eo-Anal Pouch Surgery for Ulcerative Colitis
A Guide for Patients

Zarah Perry-Woodford

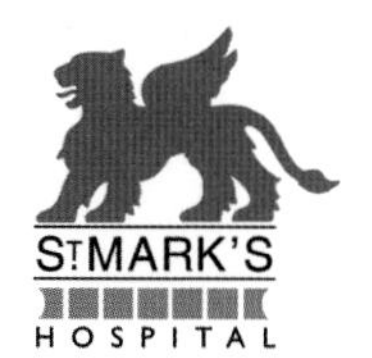

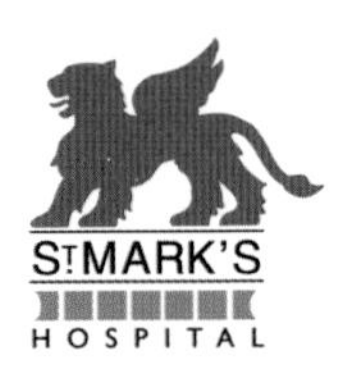

First published in the United Kingdom in 2016 by St Mark's Academic Institute, St Mark's Hospital, Northwick Park, Watford Road, Harrow, Middlesex HA1 3UJ.

Printed by Gwasg Gomer Cyf / Gomer Press Ltd, Parc Menter Llandysul, Llandysu
Ceredigion SA44 4JL.

Title: Ileo-Anal Pouch Surgery for Ulcerative Colitis – a Guide for Patients

Author: Zarah Perry-Woodford

Copy-editor, designer and illustrator: Stephen Preston

ISBN: 978-0-9935363-0-4

Chapters and sections

Foreword

Ulcerative colitis is a disease largely affecting young adults. When severe it results in consequences which may prevent normal health and functioning. Most patients can be managed by medical treatment, but over many years in a patient's life there is a chance of about a quarter to one third, that an operation will be necessary.

The surgical treatment was revolutionised in the 1970s by the introduction of the pouch operation otherwise known as restorative proctocolectomy, which enabled complete removal of the inflamed large bowel while preserving anal function thereby avoiding a permanent ileostomy (stoma).

Over the last thirty five years, the operation has changed the lives of thousands of patients and continues to do so. It is however a complex procedure and complications need careful management.

Not everybody has satisfactory bowel function. Over a ten year period the operation fails in about ten per cent of patients and an ileostomy becomes necessary, usually because of poor function associated with long-standing complications. Continuing follow-up is necessary for many patients.

When the operation was first introduced, the patient was followed by the surgeon with support from the gastroenterologist. It soon became clear, however, that neither was able to give the detailed level of care needed by patients, particularly those who were experiencing difficulties.

This led to the concept of the pouch support nurse, whose remit would be to support patients on a day-to-day basis.

The first pouch support nurse ever was appointed at St Mark's Hospital in the late 1990s and over the years many other hospitals all over the world have followed suit. The post has evolved and the pouch support nurse now plays a central role in the team, supporting the patient before, during and after the operation. The nurse is the first point of contact of patients for advice on what to do or on how to resolve a difficulty.

There are so many factors which are of concern to patients, including aspects

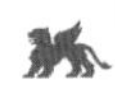

of management immediately after the operation, diet, work and sport, bowel and sexual function and liaison with the clinicians. All these have become the preserve of the pouch support nurse, who is an essential source for patients of advice and contact with the inflammatory bowel disease team.

The opportunities gained by the pouch support nurse through the direct access to patients and the experience gained in aspects of the patient's life which are not easily dealt with by the doctor, have resulted in the accumulation of a vast amount of knowledge.

In this book, Zarah Perry-Woodford has formally assessed the role of the pouch support nurse in all the various areas of activity involved. She has studied the preoperative preparation of the patient, the management of the temporary stoma resulting from restorative proctocolectomy, surgical complications and the infinitely variable management required for all the various problems that can occur over the many subsequent years.

This last aspect is one, which only someone having close contact with patients can properly deliver.

The information contained within will be of great use to patients, nurses and doctors alike. It will help health care planners to understand an area of medicine which truly represents multidisciplinary care.

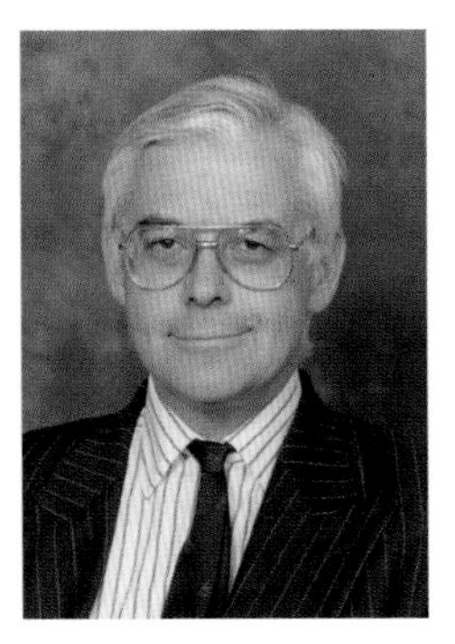

John Nicholls

MA (Cantab), MChir, FRCS(Eng), EBSQ(Coloproctology),
Hon FACS, Hon FRCP(Lond), Hon FRCSE,
Hon FRCS(Glasg), Hon ASCRS, Hon ACPGBI,
Hon ESCP, Hon BSG,
Emeritus Consultant Surgeon, St Mark's Hospital,
London Professor, Imperial College, London.

Introduction

Your surgeon has explained that you have ulcerative colitis (UC) and you need an operation as part of your treatment. This book provides information for you to understand more about the different types of operations available including necessary pre-operative and post-operative information so you can make informed decisions about your care. It will also help you understand the routine follow-up care that you will require once you leave hospital and the procedures you may have to undergo if you develop complications. This guide may need to be revisited as you embark on your surgical journey towards a pouch.

You will be given a lot of information by different health care professionals involved in your care and may not find the answers to all your questions in this book, but we hope that you will find it useful. The word 'stoma' will be used throughout this book to describe the piece of bowel which is brought out onto the abdomen and is covered by a stoma appliance or stoma bag. The word 'pouch' will describe the internal ileo-anal pouch and not the stoma bag which is sometimes also referred to as a pouch!

This book has been written by medical experts and critiqued by those living with an ileo-anal pouch. We hope it will be an asset for those who may be thinking of having surgery for UC or members of their family who may require information.

I would like to take this opportunity to thank my patients and my colleagues at St Mark's Hospital who have provided invaluable information.

If you would like further information or clarification of the content in this book it may be worthwhile to discuss these issues with your surgeon, gastroenterologist or specialist nurse. However if you would like to speak to me directly, please contact:

Zarah Perry-Woodford, lead nurse – pouch and stoma care, St Mark's Hospital
E-mail: lnwh-tr.internalpouchcare@nhs.net

 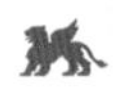

The content and images included in this book are intended for the management of patients undergoing ileo-anal pouch surgery at St Mark's Hospital and follows clinical recommendations and policies of the London North West Healthcare NHS Trust. Therefore some of the specialist services or treatment methods mentioned in this book may not be offered at your local hospital, however you may wish to discuss the treatment options discussed with your medical/surgical team.

Contributors

Lisa Allison (pouch nurse specialist)
Janindra Warusavitarne (consultant colorectal surgeon)
Stephen Wright (lead specialist practitioner)
Ellie Bradshaw (biofeedback nurse specialist)
Diane Gollagly (staff nurse, St Mark's intestinal imaging department)

Review panel

John Nicholls
Sue Clark
Janindra Warusavitarne
St Mark's Hospital stoma care
Pharmacy department
Biofeedback and radiology department
The patient panel from IA (the ileostomy and internal pouch support group)

Patient panel

Rio Dendrick
Brij Sharma
John Mullins
Preash Lad
David Danciger

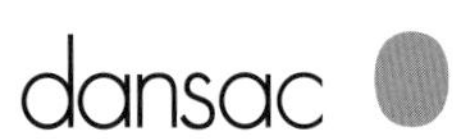

We would like to thank Dansac Ltd for their continued support of this book and their investment in nurse education and training.

About this author

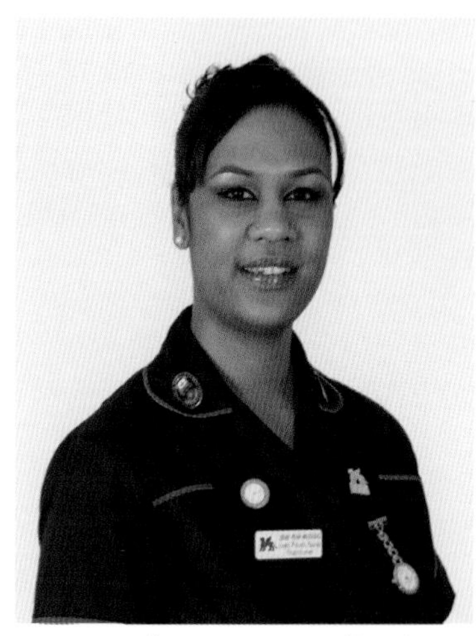
Zarah Perry-Woodford

Post qualification in 1999, I served in the Royal Air Force as a military nurse on a general/colorectal ward. In 2002, I joined St Mark's Hospital in London and worked as a senior staff nurse and then as a clinical nurse specialist in stoma care where I managed patients with stomas, ileo-anal pouches, enterocutaneous fistulae and those with intestinal failure.

Since 2005, I have worked as the lead pouch nurse practitioner providing expert care to patients with ileo-anal pouches. This team is the sole nursing service in the UK dedicated to patients with an ileo-anal pouch, providing nurse-led inpatient care, outpatient clinics and telephone advice lines. I contribute to a variety of medical and nursing journals. I also contribute to nurse education, current research and protocol development and present at national and international level. In 2014, I was promoted to lead in the stoma care team at St Mark's Hospital and work in conjunction with world renowned colorectal surgeons.

With my expertise and desire to provide high quality nursing care, it is my aim to enhance my patients' experience and offer robust support through their surgical journey.

This book is dedicated to all my patients who have inspired me by their bravery and determination to conquer ill health.

The role of the pouch nurse

The pouch nurses have an important role to play in your hospital stay. The pouch nurses at St Mark's Hospital are fully trained stoma care nurses but have extra qualifications and skills to manage patients who have an ileo-anal pouch. They usually meet you before your operation either at your appointment with the surgeon or at your preassessment appointment to give you information about the stoma and the pouch. If this is not suitable, an appointment can be arranged for another day or we will see you the day that you are admitted to the ward for surgery. In a few cases we will refer you to your local stoma care nurse who will see you before your operation.

It is important that you see a pouch nurse before your operation for pre-operative education and possibly stoma siting. Information will be given to you verbally and reinforced with this book, which can be taken home to read. On admission to hospital we are available to see you to go over information, answer questions and mark the site where the stoma will be (if this has not been done already).

Topics usually covered by the pouch nurse include:

- The role of the pouch nurse
- An explanation of the operation
- The type of stoma you will have
- Where the stoma will be on your abdomen
- Types of stoma bags (appliances)
- Recovery from surgery
- Management of the stoma
- Diet
- Lifestyle
- Follow-up care
- On-going supplies and home delivery
- Travel
- Work
- Sport
- Sexuality
- Body image

After the operation your pouch nurse will teach you how to care for the stoma. This involves learning to empty and change the stoma bag. This is done on a daily basis for you to practice and gain independence. You must demonstrate a stoma bag change independently before the pouch nurse is happy for you to be discharged home.

On discharge, if you live locally and pay your council tax to the borough of Harrow we will provide you with an out-patient appointment in one of our nurse-led clinics. If you live outside the local area then we will refer you onto the stoma care nurse who is based in your area. You can always contact us via our telephone advice line or by email even if you have a local stoma care nurse. We also provide nurse-led rapid access clinics if you require our input either before or after surgery.

The pouch nurses also have a role to play in the education of other nurses and medical staff. This involves students and junior staff spending time with the pouch nurses so they can learn how to care for patients with a stoma or pouch. Increasing the available knowledge will lead to patients receiving better care. If you would rather not be observed please mention this to your pouch nurse as we understand that some patients prefer privacy when undertaking stoma care.

We are also involved in a number of other areas such as research, development of new appliances, assisting patient support groups and presenting at national and international conferences. We may ask for your opinion to better understand your experience of pouch surgery, however our main aim is to provide you throughout your hospital stay with as much support as possible by using the skills and expertise that we have in the field of ileo-anal pouch and stoma care nursing.

Never be afraid to ask your pouch nurse questions as we are here to help you!

Preparing for surgery

The digestive system (gastrointestinal tract)

The role of the digestive system is to take food into your body, absorb the nutrients and remove harmful waste products. It is made of a hollow tube starting at the mouth and ending at the anus.

Food enters the mouth, is chewed and then enters into the stomach via the oesophagus. The food is liquidised by the acid and enzymes produced by the stomach lining and is now called 'chyme'. The chyme enters the first part of the small bowel called the duodenum where pancreatic juice (from the pancreas) is added to continue the digestive process. Digestion is completed when the chyme reaches the second part of the small bowel called the jejunum. The last part of the small bowel (the ileum) absorbs most nutrients from the digested food leaving the waste products and most of the water behind. The waste moves into the large bowel (colon) and water is absorbed here forming a solid product called faeces (stool). The faeces passes into the last part of the large intestine called the rectum which acts as a reservoir until it can be passed via the anus into the toilet.

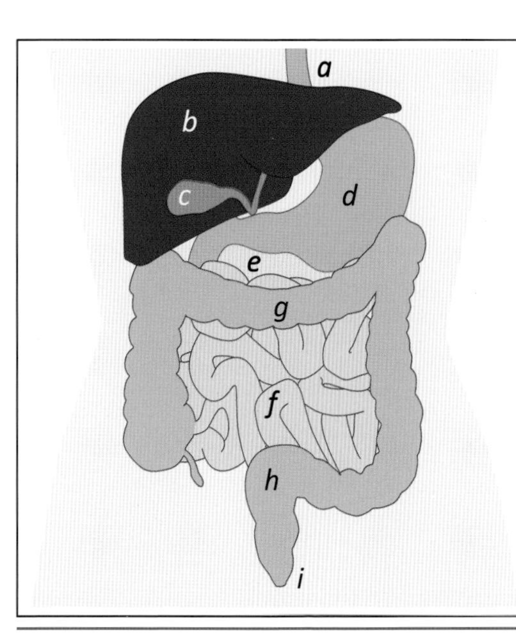

The digestive system

a. oesophagus
b. liver
c. gallbaldder
d. stomach
e. pancreas
f. small intestine
g. large intestine / colon
h. rectum
i. anus

Overview of ulcerative colitis

Ulcerative colitis (UC) is described as inflammation and ulceration of the large bowel. Symptoms can vary in severity with unpredictable periods of relapse and remission. The most common signs of UC are frequent and urgent bowel motions with bloody diarrhoea, however other symptoms may occur.

Other symptoms of UC:

- Abdominal pain and cramping
- Blood and mucous in the stool
- Diarrhoea
- Fever
- Tenesmus (feeling of incomplete emptying)
- Weight loss (or stunted growth in children)

Other symptoms outside the bowel that may occur with UC:

- Joint pain and swelling
- Mouth ulcers
- Skin rashes
- Eye complications

The cause of UC is not clear. In most situations it is treated with medical therapy but 25–30% of patients will require surgery. In UC, surgery removes the disease but the consequences can be quite significant and is therefore offered after medical treatment.

There must also be a clear diagnosis of UC before surgery, as a diagnosis of Crohn's disease is a contraindication to pouch surgery due to unacceptably high pouch failure rates. A diagnosis of indeterminate colitis can also significantly increase the risk of pouch failure. The most common reasons for surgery are:

Acute toxic colitis

This is where an acute flare-up does not respond to medical therapy. It can manifest as a combination of diarrhoea with or without blood, weight loss and pain with a general feeling of being severely unwell. In some situations there is significant risk of the colon perforating which increases the risk to any individual quite significantly with a 10% risk of death. This situation is best avoided and in acute severe colitis, careful monitoring of the individual with both serial X-rays and observation is essential. A dilated or larger than normal colon is an early sign that perforation is a significant risk.

Chronic colitis

This is where the inflammation is kept at bay by medication and there is no acute colitis but there is no major improvement despite maximum medical therapy. It usually results in a general feeling of ill health where activities of daily living are significantly affected. It can flare up into an acute attack. In addition to the general feeling of being unwell, steroid dependence is another feature of chronic colitis and often it is not possible for individuals on long term steroids to reduce the dose without increasing the symptoms of UC.

Cancer risk

In individuals with long standing colitis (usually more than 10 years of fairly active disease) there is a risk of cancer in the colon or rectum and regular colonoscopies are advised. It is always best to have a colonoscopy performed by someone who does regular colonoscopies for UC as they are much more likely to recognise a subtle change, if present.

When the colonoscopy is performed, the person performing the procedure will take multiple samples and these will be tested for precancerous cells, called dysplasia. Dysplasia can be classified into low-grade or high-grade.

If low-grade dysplasia is present then surveillance by colonoscopy can be continued in some situations but will require an indepth discussion with a gastroenterologist or surgeon about the risk and benefit of this. If high-grade dysplasia is present then the risk of a cancer developing or being present in the colon is very high and surgery is the best option.

In some situations a cancer is detected in the specimen and surgery is the option in this situation. A staging process prior to surgery will need to be performed to determine the stage of the cancer.

Surgical techniques

The traditional operation for ulcerative colitis (UC) involved opening the abdomen (tummy) and removing the large bowel through a long midline incision. Patients were hospitalised for approximately two weeks and recovery was a slow process.

The large wound was prone to breakdown and infection and meant that patients could not mobilise easily, subjecting them to further post-operative complications. From a cosmetic viewpoint open surgery was not aesthetically pleasing.

In most cases of UC, laparoscopic surgery can be performed safely but is best performed by a surgeon with significant experience in both laparoscopic surgery and surgery for UC. This technique has the benefit of a better cosmetic effect to open surgery but also has the added benefit of less pain and a shorter hospital stay with faster recovery.

Laparoscopic surgery is now considered first line treatment for bowel surgery at St Mark's Hospital and there are very few contraindications to this type of surgery.

If you have had previous operations performed by an open method, laparoscopic surgery is not impossible but may be converted to an open procedure. The risk of conversion is about 5%.

Operation choices in UC

There are three main types of operation that can be performed for ulcerative colitis:

- **Pan-proctocolectomy and permanent end stoma**
- **Subtotal colectomy and formation of a temporary end stoma**
- **Restorative proctocolectomy and formation of a temporary loop stoma (the pouch operation)**

In each operation you will have a stoma (ileostomy) formed, however, whether the stoma is permanent or temporary is determined by the type of operation chosen. The ultimate decision on the type of surgery depends on the clinical circumstances of the disease but is also an individual choice based on a comprehensive discussion with your surgeon and pouch nurse.

Any decision on the type of surgery should be made after you have sourced the required information and your questions have been clarified. The outcome of pouch surgery differs for individuals depending on your lifestyle and expectations of surgery. The pouch operation appears to be the preferred option for those patients who need surgery for UC. The attraction with this procedure is that it allows a normal route for evacuation and avoids the need for a permanent stoma. Depending on individual situations, the pouch operation can be done in one, two or three stages.

There are potential complications and associated long-term effects with any operation and thorough discussion with your surgeon and pouch nurse is essential before any decision is made. Age is not usually a barrier to pouch surgery but in those people over the age of 60 there is a risk of worse pouch function and this should be taken into consideration in the decision-making process.

1. Pan-proctocolectomy and permanent end stoma

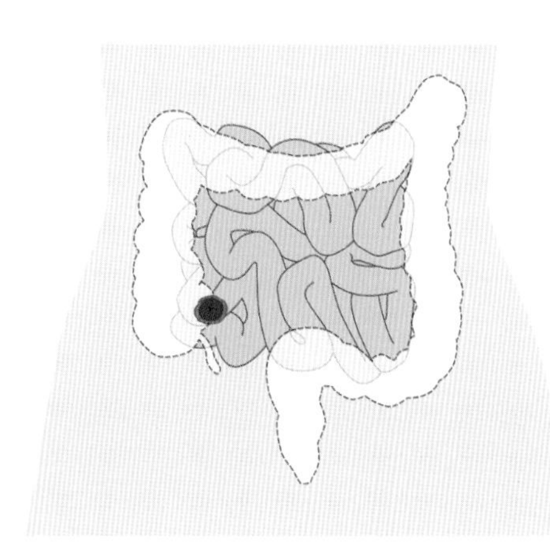

In this operation the entire colon, rectum and anus (bottom) are removed and the anus is then sewn up. The stoma is made from the end of the small bowel to create a spout which projects about 2.5 cm from the surface of the skin and the abdominal and anal wounds are sewn up.

Further surgery to create an ileo-anal pouch is now impossible. The stoma is permanent and brought out on the right side of the abdomen.

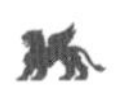

The indications for this operation are based on patient choice but some clinical situations will preside such as:

- **Presence of a very low cancer that cannot be removed without removing the anus**
- **Presence of fistula in the anus**
- **Presence of infection near the anus**
- **Weak muscles of the anus increasing the risk of faecal incontinence**

No surgical procedure is free of complications. In the case of pan-proctocolectomy with a permanent stoma there are three main problems that can occur:

a) Blockage of the intestine due to kinking

After any bowel operation, the surface of the intestine left behind becomes tacky and sticks to itself and other structures. This is known as adhesions. If the adhesions cause twisting or kinking of the intestine, then the channel down the middle can become narrowed, causing a blockage. This occurs in about 10% of cases. It may settle on its own after a few days. If it does not, an abdominal operation to un-kink the point of blockage may be necessary but unfortunately may reoccur in the future.

b) Delay in the healing of the bottom wound

This occurs in 20–40% of cases and it can take months in some cases for the wound to finally heal. For a few patients, the wound does not heal and plastic surgery may be necessary. Whilst not serious, it is an annoying complication, requiring regular dressings until healed.

c) Complications of the stoma can occur

The stoma can narrow down (stenose), fall back (retract), come out too far (prolapse) or develop a rupture (hernia). Over a five year period from the operation there is a 20–30% chance of needing another operation, usually minor, to deal with a stoma complication.

2. Subtotal colectomy and formation of an end stoma

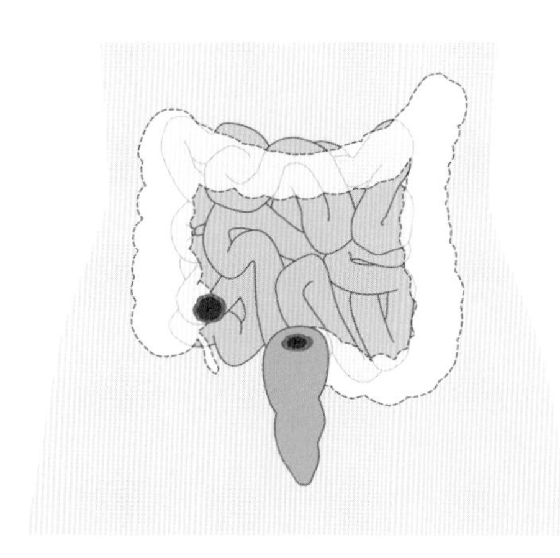

If you are very unwell (acute colitis), on high-dose steroids or have recently used Infliximab or Humira® but think you would like to have a pouch rather than a permanent stoma, it is often preferable to perform a subtotal colectomy first to remove the bulk of diseased bowel. This 'staging' of operations not only allows time for you to get better, but experience life with a stoma. This operation involves removing the colon (colectomy) leaving the rectum and anus behind.

A temporary stoma is made from the end of the small bowel to create a spout which projects about 2.5 cm from the surface of the skin and any abdominal wounds are sewn up.

Depending on how severely diseased the rectum is, the surgeon will decide whether to sew it up and leave it inside your pelvis or whether to bring it out just under the stoma or under a wound. In this case the opening in the rectum is now referred to as a mucous fistula. The mucous fistula will not heal up over time and may continue to produce mucous periodically until the rectum is removed. You may continue to pass bloodstained mucus from your anus which is not usually problematic.

The majority of the inflammation is now removed therefore recovery begins. You will have a stoma for approximately 3–9 months and be given support to decide if you want to keep the stoma or have the second operation to create a pouch and form a loop stoma in place of your end stoma. If you choose to have a pouch you will require a third operation to finally close the stoma.

3. Restorative proctocolectomy and formation of a temporary loop stoma – the pouch operation

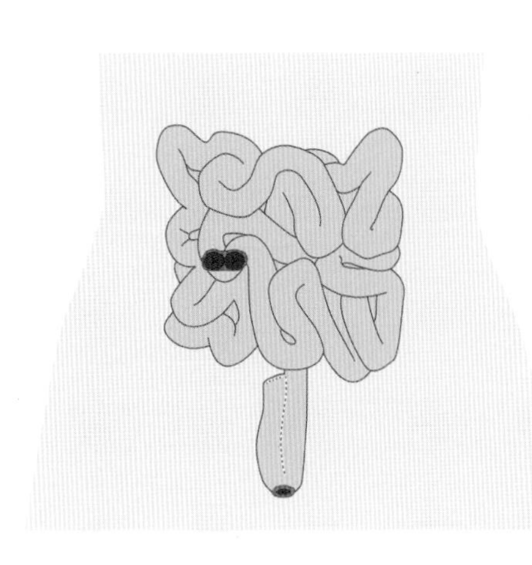

If your colitis is stable (chronic colitis), you are generally well and not on steroid medication, the pouch operation can be performed in two stages. In this operation the entire colon and rectum are removed and the end of the small bowel is folded over and opened up between the folds with a cutting stapler to form a pouch which functions as a 'new rectum'. The pouch is then connected to the anus by stitches or by a specially designed stapler.

A temporary 'loop' stoma is formed above the pouch to protect the join where the pouch is connected to the anus and reduces the risk of serious infection should there be a small leak in any of the joins.

If you previously had a subtotal colectomy you would have experienced an end stoma, however the loop stoma will look different as it appears flatter and may be larger as it is made from a loop of small bowel instead of the end. The output from a loop stoma will be of higher volume and a more liquid consistency as this stoma is further upstream (as the end of the small bowel is now made into the pouch).

Some patients require extra care with their diet and hydration and may even use anti-diarrhoeal medication to slow down the stoma output. You may still pass mucus via the pouch with a loop stoma but this is not of any concern and is not an indication of expected pouch function. The loop stoma is usually left in place for three months to allow the joins to heal. The stoma will be reversed in a separate operation before the pouch can work. In exceptional cases the pouch operation may be performed in one stage which involves removing the colon and rectum and formation of the pouch without the use of a temporary stoma. This approach has been deemed safe in some circumstances but requires a detailed conversation with the surgeon about the risks and benefits.

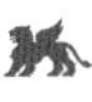

3 STAGE RPC: Subtotal colectomy and formation of end ileostomy	Proctectomy with ileo-anal pouch formation. Conversion of end ileostomy to loop ileostomy	Closure of ileostomy
2 STAGE RPC: Proctocolectomy with ileo-anal pouch and formation of loop ileostomy	Closure of ileostomy	
1 STAGE RPC: Proctocolectomy with ileo-anal pouch formation		

Overview of restorative proctocolectomy (RPC) stages

Advantages and disadvantages of pouch surgery

Contemplating surgery can be a daunting experience for most people.

The best way to be reassured that you are doing the right thing for you is to consider the following:

- Get as much information about the operation as possible from reliable sources
- Speak or meet other people who have undergone similar experiences
- Join a support group – see the list at the back of this book
- Research the hospital and what they offer before, during and after the operation
- Know your surgeon, meet them and ask questions
- Meet your pouch nurse

The aim of pouch surgery is to restore bowel continuity and hopefully continence, therefore avoiding the need for a permanent stoma. However you do not have to have a pouch or feel pressured into having one as some people actually choose to keep their stoma. What is important is you choose an option that you are comfortable with. Many people choose to have a pouch because it fits in with their lifestyle and enhances their body image. It is very difficult for most people to decide which operation to have especially if they have never had a stoma or a pouch before. There are advantages and disadvantages to every surgical intervention. To help you make an informed choice the advantages and disadvantages involved in pouch surgery have been listed below. Overall, most people have an excellent outcome following pouch surgery.

Advantages of the ileo-anal pouch

1. Removal of disease

With a competent and experienced surgeon, disease is removed and the impending cancer risk significantly reduced. There have been many studies assessing the cancer risk within the ileo-anal pouch and conclude that cancer in the pouch is rare and therefore quality of life is immediately improved.

If you have been undergoing invasive and uncomfortable testing to track your disease course or using high-dose steroids or other drugs to combat the effects of your illness, you may find that the ileo-anal pouch offers widespread relief and provides some form of a 'normal' life.

2. Eliminates the initial need for a permanent stoma

In some people who have an aversion to a permanent stoma, the ileo-anal pouch offers a temporary stoma which is reversed in a few months. This gives you an idea of what stoma care involves in case the pouch fails and you are presented with the decision to return to a stoma.

3. Patient choice

The pouch operation is an 'elective' procedure, which means you can choose to have a pouch if you want one. The pouch operation is seen as a cosmetic choice as you do not need to have one in order to remove your disease.

You do not have to agree to pouch surgery immediately and are given the chance to research the options especially if your disease is controlled or you are not at high-risk of cancer in the rectum. Some people choose to complete their family or career interests before committing to pouch surgery.

4. Normal diet can be achieved

Normal diet can be introduced within a couple of weeks following closure of the stoma. Most people have a general idea of the sorts of foods that may have upset their stoma function and this remains the same in the early days after stoma closure. Small, regular and low fibre meals are paramount in promoting an acceptable pouch function in the early days.

You are encouraged to experiment with different foods and monitor your pouch function. It is also worth remembering that the pouch will need to undergo some degree of training to ensure good function and this can be enhanced with a nutritious, regular diet pattern.

You can also discuss this further with your pouch nurse. Some people may require input from a dietitian if they fail to gain weight after surgery.

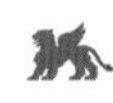

5. Sexual function may be improved

Some people have found that sexual function is improved following pouch surgery. This may be related to the improved quality of life and body image from the removal of the stoma and associated reservations. Sperm banking and egg harvesting is not deemed necessary unless you have had radiotherapy or some types of chemotherapy pre-operatively.

6. Research and development

The ileo-anal pouch has been around since 1978 and is now seen as the 'gold standard' operation for most people requiring surgery for UC. This established operation is offered to most people. If, however, your local surgeon does not feel competent to perform surgery themselves, they may refer you to a specialist centre for treatment.

Even at large, specialist centres we are still trying to find out more about pouches and how we can make things better. Research and development is ongoing and you may be asked to give your views on the surgery or be instrumental in finding new treatment options. Being involved with research and development is not compulsory.

7. Laparoscopic surgery

Most people can now opt for laparoscopic pouch surgery commonly described as 'keyhole' surgery. This involves smaller incisions, faster recovery times and shorter hospital stays. Not all hospitals perform laparoscopic surgery and it is best to get a recommendation so that you can research your surgeon intensively.

8. Improved quality of life

In most people who opt for a pouch, the advantage of not living with a permanent stoma has benefits in terms of their lifestyle, self-esteem and sexual function. Most people report an improved quality of life.

Disadvantages of the ileo-anal pouch

1. Multiple operations

The pouch operation is usually more commonly performed in two operations but in some cases, three. This may take anywhere from six months to two years before completion and many people may have to put their life and their families on hold while they deal with hospital admissions and recovery time.

2. Longer operating times

Laparoscopic 'keyhole' operations take approximately 2–3 hours longer in theatre than open (traditional) surgery. This may be a concern if you cannot tolerate general anaesthetics for long periods of time.

3. Usually only done in larger specialist centres

The operation is increasingly being performed in district general hospitals as more surgeons become competent in the surgical technique, however specialist centres still hold the expert teams and are able to offer better follow-up and support than smaller general hospitals. For many people this necessitates long journeys and disruptions from family or work. You may also find it hard if your family can not travel to visit you as often.

4. Complications of pouch surgery

As with any operation, complications may occur in the early or late phase after surgery. These complications can be treated with a variety of means such as drug therapy (antibiotics), further investigations, diagnostic imaging or possible return to theatre for dilation or examinations. As current research evolves the diagnosis of complications is becoming easier as is the long term management of these problems.

5. No guarantee on length of pouch success

Unfortunately some pouches fail over time. Failure is defined as the need to remove the pouch or establish a stoma indefinitely. Like most things, people find that their pouch works less effectively the longer they have had them. There is no guarantee how long your pouch will last but you can be offered help and advice on managing a failing pouch. Pouch success is influenced by individual perceptions of acceptable pouch function and quality of life. Therefore what may be seen as poor pouch function for one person may not seem such a problem to another.

6. Normal pouch function is not the same as the healthy population

Stool frequency ranges from between 4–8 times in every 24 hours. Some people need to evacuate the pouch at least once at night. Most people can control the urge to defaecate for over half an hour and urgency is uncommon. Some people report nocturnal seepage. Occasionally it may be necessary to wear a sanitary pad for peace of mind. You should be made aware in the pre-operative stage that pouch frequency may increase from your experience of what is normal and you will have to make changes to incorporate this into your daily life. Most people find their pouch function is better when they are distracted, such as at work or commuting. You will never be able to empty the pouch only once a day.

7. Inability to pass wind

Most patients cannot pass wind from their pouch unless sitting on the toilet or lying down. This is common and not usually a problem. Sometimes a build up of trapped wind can become uncomfortable but is remedied once you empty your pouch.

8. Managing your expectations

Unfortunately a pouch can never work as well as a healthy rectum. The people who have realistic expectations about their pouch usually manage much better and are able to deal with possible complications. It is also important to plan carefully if you are going abroad or doing something different from your routine as your pouch may behave differently.

9. Sexual function changes

Most people who undergo pouch surgery are young and sexually active and therefore very concerned about their sexual function following surgery. The risk of sexual dysfunction is lower if you have an experienced surgeon. It is vital you discuss your individual situation with your surgeon or pouch nurse before committing to pouch surgery.

Sexual function in females

There is approximately a 50% reduction in fertility in women after open pouch surgery but this risk is much less with modern laparoscopic 'keyhole' approaches. This is mainly due to the scar tissue in your abdomen that may stop the egg moving down the fallopian tube to meet the sperm. It does not mean you cannot have a baby but it may take considerably longer to conceive or that you may need help.

Some couples find in vitro fertilization (IVF) successful. It is therefore advisable to establish in the pre-operative phase the risk to yourself of reduction in fertility and the consequences of needing IVF. Some women report painful intercourse and should wait until they feel ready to resume a sexual relationship. During pregnancy there is often an increase in pouch frequency, urgency, seepage and incontinence, however this usually returns to the prenatal state following delivery.

Sexual function in men

There is a significant risk of male sexual dysfunction, such as erectile dysfunction, absence of ejaculation (dry orgasm) or retrograde ejaculation after pelvic surgery. Most of these complications are short-lived and return to normal by themselves. If the symptoms persist you will be referred to a specialist urology team for further investigation.

10. Annual follow-up

Most large centres now discharge you back into the care of your GP. However some people are followed-up annually, depending on if they have a history of rectal cancer before pouch surgery, chronic pouchitis or have a liver condition called primary sclerosing cholangitis (PSC). For some people who have endured years of pre-operative screening this may appear as a daunting, life-long task after surgery, however many people view this as a necessity for general peace of mind.

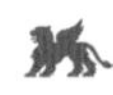

Preparing for and during surgery

It is usual to be admitted on the day of surgery for an elective operation. It is best that all major questions, discussions and stoma siting occur before you are admitted to hospital so you have time to understand the surgery before the operation. This is not always possible in the emergency setting but it is best to have as many discussions with the surgeon, pouch support nurse and members of support groups prior to surgery if possible.

You may be given a carbohydrate-rich drink to have six hours before the operation (normally at home) prior to coming to hospital. You should also have had an injection the night before surgery to prevent you developing a blood clot, also known as deep vein thrombosis (DVT). These injections usually continue after the operation until you are moving around independently. After the surgery you will follow an enhanced recovery program which is designed to improve the recovery process and minimise the impact of surgery.

Stoma siting

It is important to be sited before your operation so the stoma is placed in the best possible position. A mark will be placed on your abdomen where the surgeon will make the stoma during the operation. The pouch nurse will use her knowledge to guide and advise you on the best position. Sometimes the position the pouch nurse thinks is best is not the position you would like the stoma to be placed in.

The pouch nurse will ask you a number of questions about the clothing you wear. The belt line is avoided as much as possible. You will be asked questions about your lifestyle and how the stoma will fit into your daily activities. The shape of your abdomen will be viewed in different positions such as lying, sitting and standing, as your abdomen changes shape when you move. You will be asked to cough or sit up while a hand is placed on your abdomen to feel your abdominal muscles. This is so the stoma is placed in a strong band of muscles for support. It is important that you can see the stoma site, as you will be caring for the stoma at home.

Old scars or skin folds are avoided as these can cause problems with leakages if the stoma is too close. Sometimes creases are marked in the eventuality that the surgeon may have to move the stoma site slightly. The surgeon rarely

e initial site is placed on piece of tape. This can be oved around the abdomen til the correct position is hieved. Creases and skin folds e avoided.

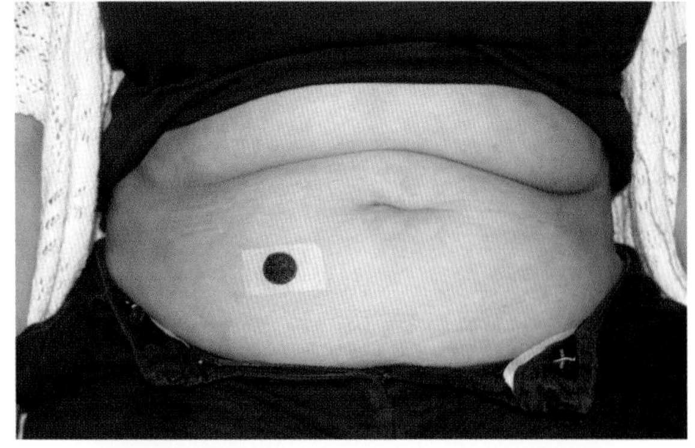

e final site is marked with an delible pen and covered with waterproof plaster.

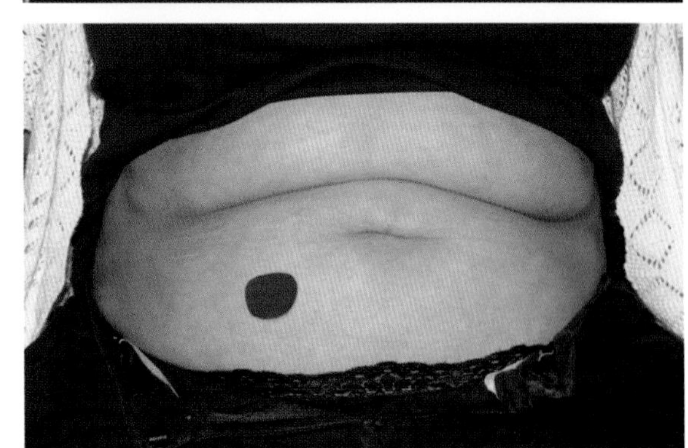

e may stick the stoma bag on u to tell if it is in a safe and mfortable position.

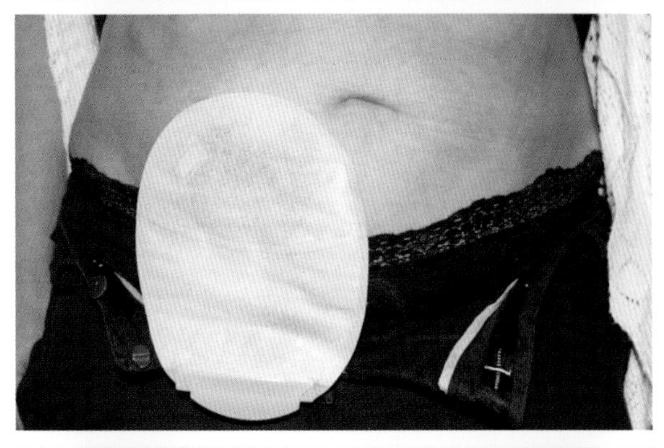

ith a low waistband, the top the bag usually appears ove the belt line.

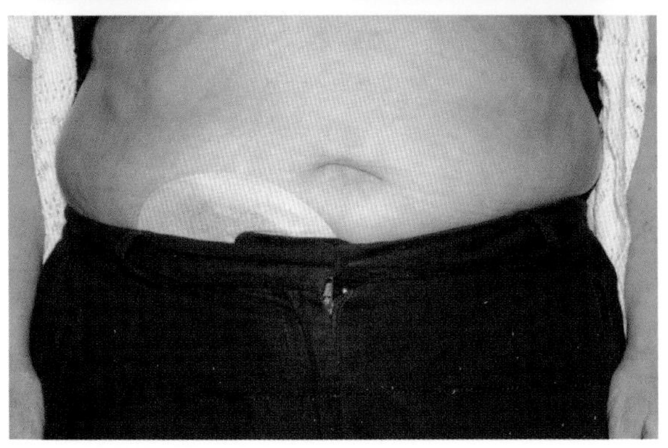

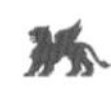

moves the agreed site and will only do so if it becomes necessary during surgery. If there are any concerns, the pouch nurse may mark both sides of your abdomen but you will only have one stoma. You will be asked to sign a consent form agreeing to the stoma site as you must understand why you have been sited. Even though the stoma is temporary it needs to be in the right position for you.

Day of surgery

You will be given a theatre gown and stockings to prevent a DVT. You must wear your stockings until you are fully mobile. Post-operative pain will be controlled using either an epidural or a patient controlled analgesia (PCA), this will be discussed when you see the anaesthetist on the day of surgery. An epidural uses a small plastic tube in your back to deliver painkillers. A PCA uses a button which goes into a drip in your arm or hand which you can push to help reduce pain. You may also be sited by the pouch nurse if this has not already been done. You will then be taken to the operating theatre.

During the operation

The surgery for a pouch can take up to six hours. During this time you will be asleep under an anaesthetic and the fluids and medications will be given by a drip into your arm. A catheter is inserted into your bladder to measure your urine output. The catheter will remain for several days after surgery. In some situations a tube will be placed in your stomach via the nose, called a nasogastric tube. This is usually inserted while you are asleep and is removed after surgery. In about 10–15% of situations it may need to be reinserted if an ileus occurs after surgery. The anaesthetist may give a single dose of antibiotics to reduce the risk of infection after surgery.

Day 0 post-operatively

Your first recollection is usually in the recovery room. In the recovery room you will be connected to a drip in your arm to provide fluids, a catheter in the bladder to drain the urine and a button connected to a machine that can deliver pain killers as required (PCA).

In addition further pain relief is given in the recovery room. Some regular pain relief is then continued on the ward and the PCA or epidural is maintained in the first 24–48 hours or longer if required to deal with pain that is not controlled by regular painkillers. Fluids by mouth are also allowed in the recovery room unless stated otherwise by the surgeon. Diet is started as soon as possible and this may be on the same day as your operation.

Day 1 post-operatively

Soon after the surgery you will be encouraged to sit out of bed and walk with the aid of a physiotherapist and by yourself over the next few days. You will be encouraged to walk 60 metres on four separate occasions, and if you can, remain sitting out of bed for six hours. Any intravenous fluids (drip) which are running will be stopped. If a urinary catheter (a tube in your bladder) has been inserted in theatre this may also be removed.

The epidural or PCA will continue but you will also be given other painkillers in the form of tablets to help reduce pain. A normal diet is encouraged and two litres of oral fluids including high calorie drinks. Your pouch nurse will begin teaching you how to look after your stoma as soon as you feel able and this is usually on the first day after your operation.

Day 2 post-operatively

Painkillers delivered by epidural or PCA are usually stopped on day two and suitable tablet and liquid painkillers which can be taken by mouth will be given. You will be encouraged to wash and dress in your own clothes.

A normal diet will be encouraged including high calorie drinks. Walking will be encouraged as on day one. Stoma care teaching will continue. You should now be independently emptying the bag. Teaching will continue with changing and emptying the stoma bag.

Day 3 post-operatively

By day three you should be feeling better, eating and drinking normally, walking around the ward area, with pain adequately controlled with oral painkillers. Stoma care teaching will continue and once you are confident in caring for your own stoma you will be able to go home. If the pouch nurse cannot see you, for example over the weekend, the bag will be changed with a ward nurse. Every time the bag is changed, it is an opportunity to learn how to do your stoma care. It is vital you can do your stoma care otherwise your discharge will be delayed.

Checks are made to ensure that you and your family are confident with discharge from day three onwards and depending on which operation you have had.

Stoma care

Appliances

The stoma care department at St Mark's Hospital has many different types of appliances available for you to use. The pouch nurse will give you advice on suitable appliances that you can choose. Sometimes the type of stoma, volume of output, where the stoma is situated and lifestyle may limit your choice of appliance. Appliances are available in one-piece and two-piece systems.

They are also available in different sizes mini, midi and maxi. Your pouch nurse will discuss the advantages and disadvantages of each system in greater depth when you are choosing an appliance. You may also wish to do this when you are discharged with your local stoma care nurse. Some patients with a loop stoma may benefit from using a convex bag but this will be discussed before discharge.

Ileostomy appliance (stoma bag)

As the output from an ileostomy will always be loose (porridge consistency) the appliance you use will have a Velcro® fastening on the end to close it. This will allow you to empty the appliance as it fills up during the day, without having to remove the whole appliance.

Some examples of drainable stoma appliances used with the ileo-anal pouch patients who have a stoma are shown overleaf:

1. An opaque midi appliance (front and back)
2. An opaque maxi appliance
3. A clear appliance used post-operation for 1–2 days (front and back)
4. Two different sized convex appliances used mainly with a loop ileostomy
5. A convex appliance in profile

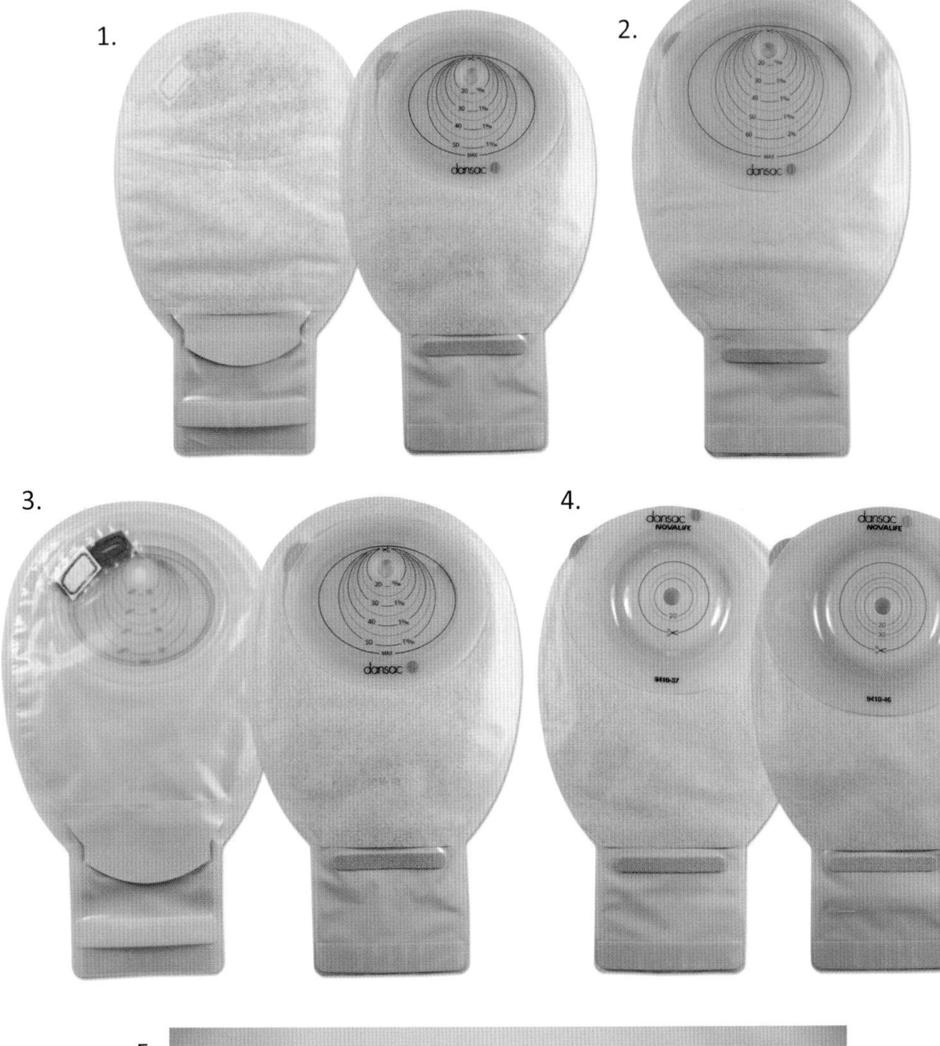
1.
dansac
2.
dansac
3.
dansac
4.
dansac
NOVALIFE
9410-37
dansac
NOVALIFE
9410-46

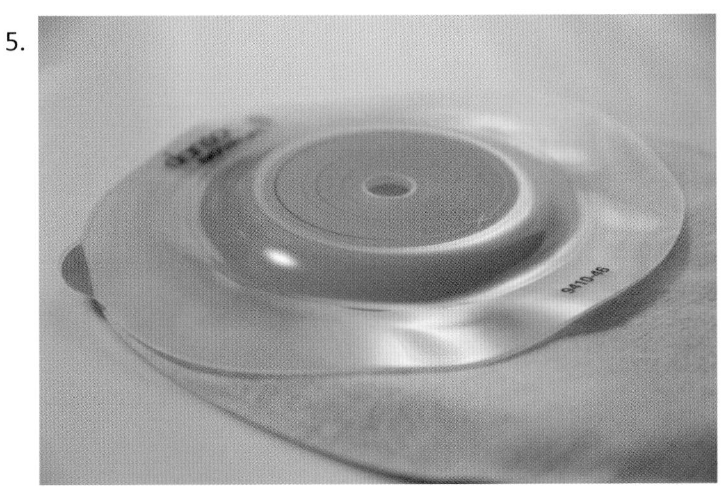
5.
9410-46

Other accessory products

Sometimes the pouch nurse may use accessory products in order to protect the skin around the stoma or help the appliance stay on for longer. These are in addition to your usual appliance and may not be required long-term. Accessory products may be in the form of tapes, wipes, sprays, powders or pastes. You do not always need an accessory product but will be guided by your pouch nurse who will advise you on which ones are suitable for you and how often you need to use them for. The pictures here shows some commonly used accessories.

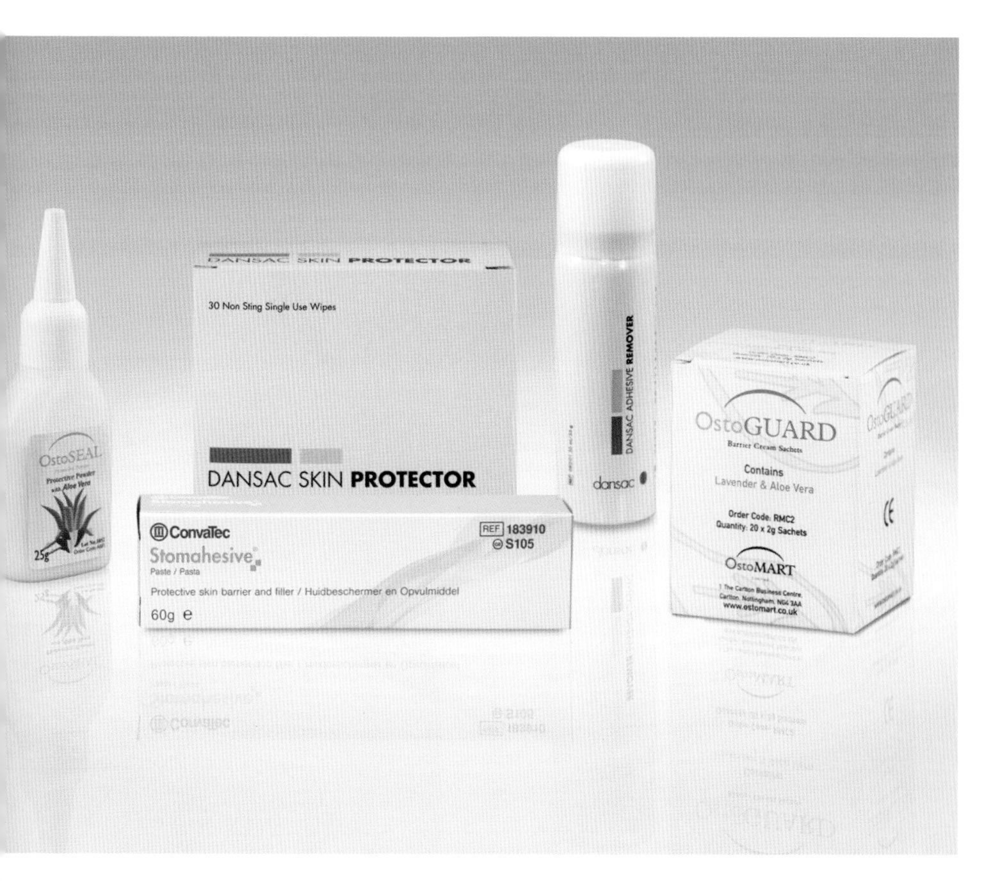

Pictured: OstoSeal Protective Powder, Dansac Adhesive Remover (30 non-sting single use wipes), Dansac Adhesive Remover spray, OstoGuard Barrier Cream Sachets, ConvaTec Stomahesive protective skin barrier and filler.

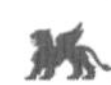

Appliance change procedure

1. Remover spray

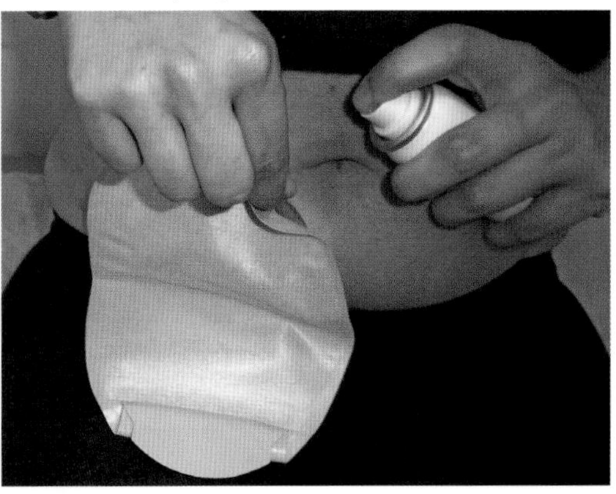

2. Peel off appliance

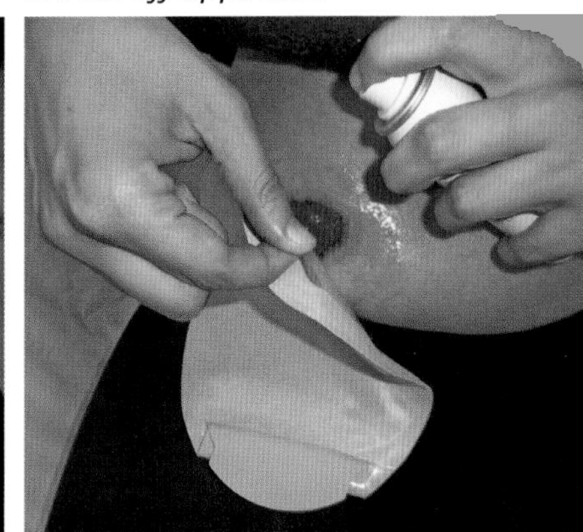

3. Clean skin

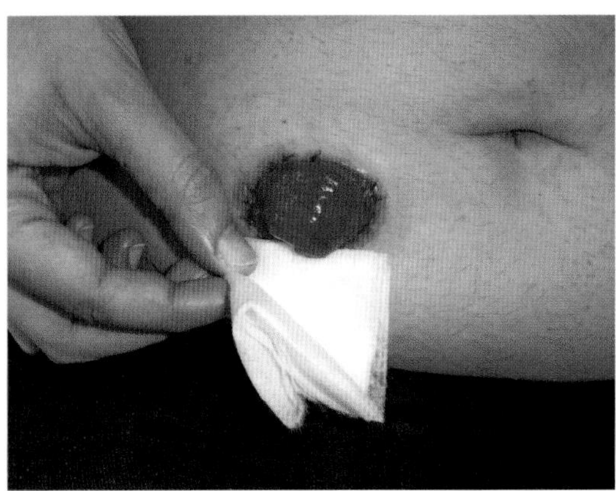

4. Measure stoma

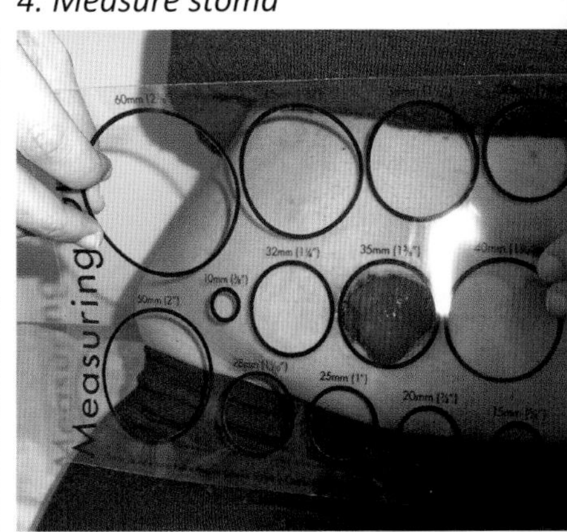

5. Cut flange

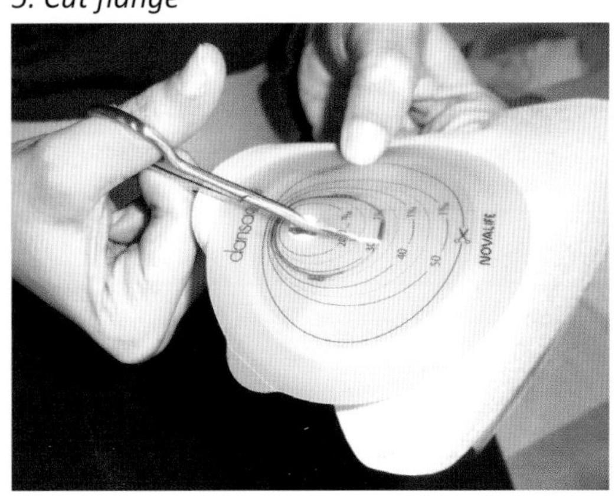

6. Cut flange

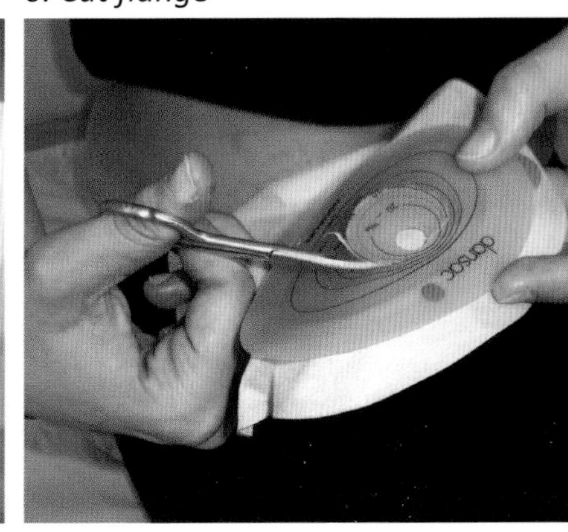

Your pouch nurse will assist you until you are confident to change the bag by yourself.

nove backing

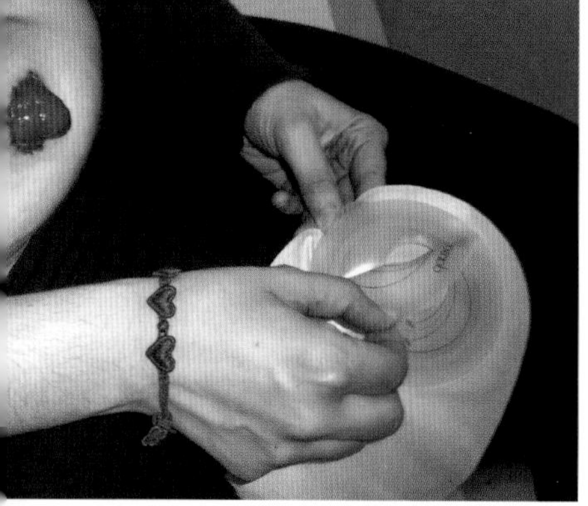

8. Position appliance

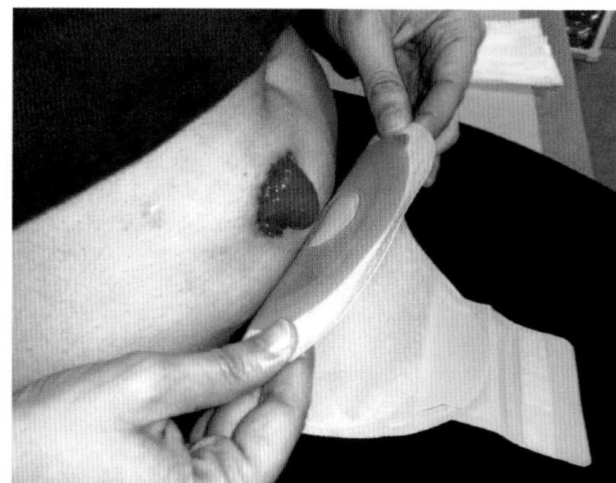

ition appliance

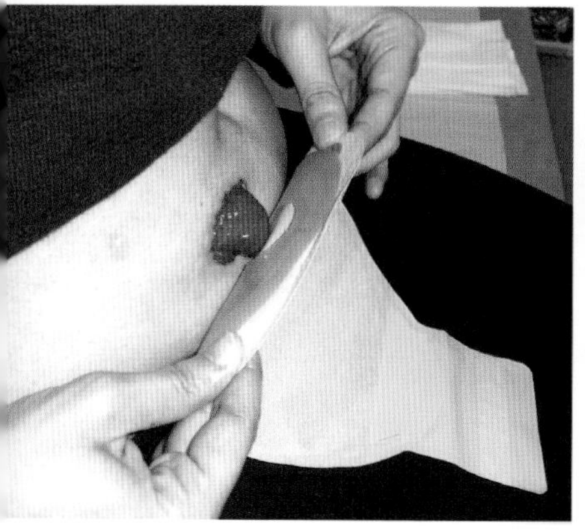

10. Roll up bag

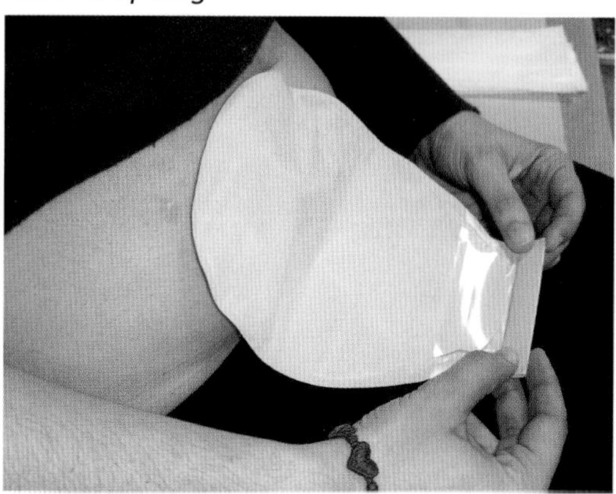

cure opening

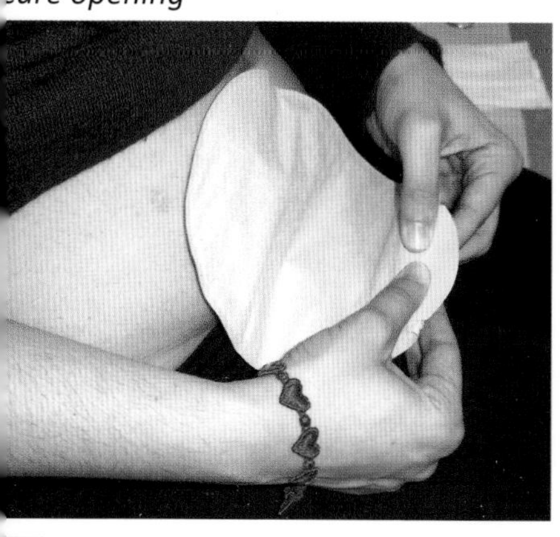

12. Appliance in place

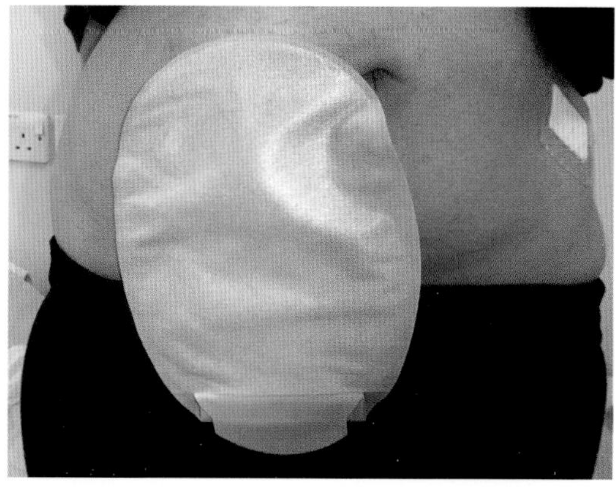

Stoma complications

Some people may have a stoma-related complication at some time after surgery ranging from minor skin irritations to more challenging complications. It is important to remember that having a stoma-related problem does not mean that you have done anything wrong when looking after your stoma. Your pouch nurse will be able to help you to manage most problems.

Wound infection

Sometimes a wound infection can develop a few days after the operation. If you have had open surgery and there is a wound running down the centre of your abdomen a wound infection can sometimes cause problems with positioning of the stoma appliance. If this is the case the pouch nurse can help with offsetting the baseplate so that it does not adhere to the wound. Wound clips are usually removed approximately 10–14 days following surgery but if an infection develops, some of the clips may be removed before this time to allow the area to drain. If the surgeon thinks it is appropriate you may be started on antibiotics. Dressings are usually advised when you are in hospital but if everything is clean and dry when you go home they can be removed. If there are any problems, the wound can be monitored by the district nurse or practice nurse once discharged.

Where you have had laparoscopic or keyhole surgery, the port sites are usually covered with a tiny dressing or glue. The glue seals the sites and comes off by itself over a few weeks. If one of the port sites is under the baseplate of the stoma appliance it can sometimes become irritated and the glue comes off earlier. If this is the case the pouch nurse will advise how best to manage the port site when caring for your stoma. If you are worried that any of your wounds or ports sites have become more painful, red, hardened or start oozing fluid please seek medical advice. A stoma is not a wound and therefore does not get infected, however, the skin around the stoma may become inflamed and you will need advice from your pouch nurse.

Ileus

Food passes through the bowel with a regular contraction and relaxation of the muscles known as peristalsis. When the bowel has been operated on it is common for peristalsis to stop occurring and this causes fluids and food to stop moving through the bowel. This can lead to the abdomen becoming bloated and you feeling nauseous. The stoma can also sometimes stop producing fluid as nothing is able to pass through. If you start to vomit then it is commonly advised that a nasogastric tube is inserted in order to relieve the pressure on the abdomen. A member of the nursing staff would insert a thin plastic tube up through the nose, down the back of the throat and into the stomach. The tube would be secured to the nose with a piece of tape and then a drainage bag attached to the other end. This enables the stomach contents to drain into the bag and relieve some of the bloated feeling and nausea. Intravenous fluids would also be needed during this period in order to keep hydrated. The bowel will start functioning properly again but it can sometimes take a few days for everything to settle. After a period of the bowel not functioning properly the stoma sometimes becomes overactive and a high output stoma bag needs to be used for a few days.

Blockage

A partial blockage may occur any time after surgery and usually this is caused by a food bolus (undigested food) stopping the natural movement through the stoma. Sometimes the bowel may twist slightly (volvulus) causing abdominal distension, nausea and pain. It is advised that you stop eating and drink fluids only for a few hours to attempt to 'flush' the obstruction through. It may be wise to drink a couple glasses of water quickly to help move things along. Some people find a brisk walk, abdominal massage or relaxing in a warm bath may help. If, however, you do become more bloated, the pain increases or you begin to vomit, you must seek medical advice immediately!

Excoriated skin

Excoriated skin is caused by the output coming into contact with the skin around the stoma. Reasons for this can be if the stoma bag is cut too big or the stoma has reduced in size and has not been measured properly. Occasionally it may be because the output has become more watery and it is getting underneath the baseplate. It can be treated by simply resizing the stoma or reassessing the skin around the stoma. Sometimes accessories may be used such as powders, pastes or skin barriers which your pouch nurse can advise you on. On some occasions your pouch nurse may suggest you use medication which will slow down the output from your stoma.

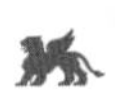

Blood

Blood is normal when wiping the stoma with soft wipes as the bowel has a lot of blood vessels. You should only be concerned if the blood appears to be coming from inside the stoma and is starting to make the output in the bag bloody. Please contact your pouch nurse or a medical professional if you are worried.

Mucocutaneous separation

Mucocutaneous separation is where the stoma is under some degree of tension causing the skin edges to pull away from the stoma. This normally happens in the first few weeks after surgery and is quite common. It can be very superficial at skin level or deeper down to the fatty layer of the skin. Your pouch nurse will assess the separation and advise you on treatment. This may include using powder or paste.

Retraction

Retraction is where the stoma is under tension and is pulled back into the abdomen. This can happen immediately after surgery when the stoma is created under tension or over a long period of time such as if you gain weight. You may find your appliance starts to leak frequently and causes your skin to become sore and excoriated. There are varying degrees of retraction and a number of treatment options. If you think your stoma is retracting then contact your pouch nurse who will assess you and advise on treatment to manage this problem. In many cases simply changing to a different type of appliance will solve the problem. In a few instances this problem may become unmanageable and surgery may be required to refashion the stoma and correct the problem.

Stenosis

Stenosis occurs when the scar tissue round the stoma causes the stoma to become narrow. The scar tissue may have developed after mucocutaneous separation or the abdominal opening being too tight. If you think your stoma is becoming tighter or narrower then contact your pouch nurse. You may be advised to dilate your stoma, using a dilator to keep it open, or you may be referred back to your surgeon to refashion your stoma under an anaesthetic.

Prolapsed stoma

A prolapsed stoma is caused when more bowel moves out of the abdomen. A prolapse may be due to inadequate fixing of the stoma to the abdominal wall at the time of surgery. A prolapse can be managed by using a larger appliance to accommodate the extra bowel. In other cases it may be possible to manually reduce the prolapse when you are lying flat. It is important for you to make sure that the prolapsed bowel does not become damaged or change colour. If this occurs please contact your pouch nurse.

High output

High output from your stoma may result in acute dehydration. If you have had an end stoma before you may notice that your loop stoma output is more liquid and that you may have to empty your bag more often. This can happen with a loop stoma because this stoma is higher up in the bowel (closer to your stomach) than your end stoma was. This means your food and drink have less time in the bowel to be absorbed and are lost quicker than in a stoma at the end of the bowel. It is advised you drink at least one and a half to two litres of fluid a day and add salt to your diet. You may be advised to use medication to slow down the bowel function.

Parastomal hernia

A parastomal hernia is the bulging of the intestine under the skin through the opening in the muscle wall where your stoma has been brought through. A parastomal hernia may cause pain and discomfort around the stoma and some people report a dragging or heavy sensation. Some hernias may become strangulated and cause an obstruction in the bowel.

Depending on the size of your hernia there are a number of ways that it can be managed. Abdominal supports can be used to disguise and support the weight. These may be in the form of a belt or underwear and are available on prescription. Your pouch nurse will arrange for you to be measured and order you one. The hernia may cause problems with your appliance, for example, the bulge can cause your bags to lift off and leak. In some cases the hernia may become unmanageable or cause frequent obstructions. In these situations your surgeon may decide to operate in order to repair the hernia.

 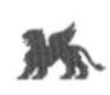

There are some predisposing factors for a hernia. They include:

- Increased age
- Multiple operations
- Wound infections
- Heavy lifting
- Obesity
- Steroid therapy
- Malnutrition
- Wide abdominal defect
- Peristomal infection
- Sited outside rectus muscle
- Poor abdominal wall support
- Construction defects
- Urinary retention
- Increased abdominal pressure e.g. coughing
- Diminished muscle tone
- Collagen defects/disorder

Allergies

Allergies to the baseplate of the stoma appliances are quite rare but can sometimes occur if you have very sensitive skin. If an allergy occurs you will see a red ring all around the edge of your stoma – the shape of the baseplate. If this happens your pouch nurse will help you find another appliance that suits your skin.

Mucous fistula

A mucous fistula is formed when the end of the rectum is left open at the top and brought out usually along the side of the stoma. It is not always visible. The rectum will naturally produce mucus (which may be bloodstained) and this will either be passed from the anus or come up through the mucous fistula. The stoma appliance may need to be cut slightly larger near the mucous fistula to allow the mucus to drain into the bag as opposed to underneath the baseplate which will cause the appliance to leak. Some surgeons attach the end of the rectum to the underside of one of the laparoscopic port sites or to a slightly larger wound above the pubic area.

If either of these areas begin to go hard or red it could mean that there is a build-up of mucus and that it may need to be drained. If you are concerned you must contact your GP or pouch team.

Dietary requirements with a stoma

Dietary requirements will vary from one person to another and will depend on your individual lifestyle and eating patterns. These recommendations serve only as a guide and must be tailored to individual need.

Foods to include and those to avoid immediately after surgery

Include (soluble fibre)	Avoid (insoluble fibre)
White bread or half wholemeal varieties	Wholegrain or wholemeal products
White rice / pasta	Raw, unpeeled fruit
Refined cereals, e.g. Corn Flakes®	Raw vegetables
Peeled or mashed potatoes	Dried fruit or berries
Peeled, canned or cooked fruit	Dried beans and pulses
Well cooked or minced meat	Unshelled lentils
Fish	Coconut
Eggs	Spicy foods
Cheese	Nuts
Soup (strained)	Seeds
Salty biscuits, crisps and snacks	Skins on fruit and vegetables
Smooth juice and squash	Juice with pulp
Bananas	Undercooked meat or meat with gristle

One of the primary roles of the colon is to absorb fluids. Though your body will adapt to living without a colon after stoma formation you will lose fluid and some salt through the stoma so it is important that dietary precautions are taken in the first few weeks after surgery. You will also need to drink approximately 1.5–2 litres (8–10 glasses) of fluid a day to make up for the fluid loss and to avoid becoming dehydrated.

It is essential that you also include salt in your diet. This means cooking with salt, adding salt to your food or eating foods and snacks that contain salt. You need about a teaspoon of salt per day after stoma forming surgery. If you have been advised to avoid salt for a medical reason, such as high blood pressure, you may wish to discuss this further with your pouch nurse, GP or surgeon as it is likely you will still need to increase your salt intake to prevent dehydration.

After surgery you will be allowed to eat a light, low residue diet as soon as you are able to, which can be the same day as the operation. After surgery it is important to have a balanced diet in order to promote healing and gain weight if necessary.

Once you have an established stoma (after six weeks) you can reintroduce most foods. Your dietary requirements will differ according to your personal situation and lifestyle but with an established stoma you may begin to enjoy foods you probably avoided when you were unwell.

New stoma (the first six weeks)

In the first six weeks after stoma-forming surgery, some adjustments may be required to your diet to prevent a bowel obstruction, excessive odour, wind, pain or a high output.

Most people may find it easier to eat small frequent meals and snacks rather than three full meals a day. It is advisable to eat a low residue/low fibre diet therefore avoiding insoluble fibre.

Insoluble fibre speeds up the transit time of the bowel causing food to move through more quickly and may cause a high liquid output from your stoma. This in turn means you may become dehydrated as you will empty your bag more often. Insoluble fibre can also cause wind (pain) and potentially block the bowel in the early days.

Foods that affect stoma output

Thicken	Thin	Obstruct	Wind
Smooth peanut butter	Green leafy vegetables	Nuts	Green vegetables (leafy)
Tapioca pudding	High fibrous foods	Pith	High fibrous foods
Mashed potato	Baked beans	Raw vegetables	Peas, beans
Bananas	Fried foods	Raw fruit	Lentils
White rice	Spicy foods	Mushrooms	Eggs, strong chees
White pasta	Chocolate	Coconut	Bran
White bread	Fruit juices	Fruit skins	Broccoli, sprouts
Toast	Caffeine	Peas	Onions
Boiled milk	Alcohol	Lettuce	Asparagus
Flat lemonade	Milk	Coleslaw	Cabbage
Grated apple	Spinach	Pineapple	Fruit skins
Apple sauce	Raw fruit	Seeds	Dried fruits
Yoghurt	Cabbage	Brown bread	Nuts, seeds
Cheese	Broccoli	Brown pasta	Chewing gum
Marshmallows		Dried fruit	Rich, creamy food
Jelly babies		Sweetcorn	Fried, fatty food
		Celery	Mushrooms
		Tough meats	Sweetcorn
		Shrimp	Baked beans
		Lobster	Cauliflower
			Cucumber
			Garlic, mustard
			Peanut butter

Stoma diet

If you are accustomed to eating a high fibre diet you may find that you are able to tolerate insoluble fibre earlier than six weeks after surgery. It is still advised that you avoid most insoluble fibre and this can be achieved by peeling or shelling pulses and vegetables.

You must also remember to chew everything thoroughly as this will make the foods you have chosen easier to digest. If you fancy foods that may be high in fibre, try a small amount and see how they affect you. If you feel bloated or uncomfortable it is probably wise to avoid them for a bit longer and try them again at a later date. It is also suggested you reintroduce foods slowly to avoid side effects such as an obstruction or high output. If you continue to suffer ill effects with certain foods it is probably best to avoid them altogether.

Established stoma (six weeks following surgery)

After six weeks, you may try introducing a more varied diet, with food from all the major food groups including fibre.

There are two types of fibre, insoluble and soluble:

1. Insoluble fibre bulks your stool and increases the movement of stool through your digestive tract, therefore increasing your output.
2. Soluble fibre dissolves in water to form a gel-like substance therefore slowing your output. Reducing insoluble fibre and increasing soluble fibre in your diet may reduce and thicken your stoma output.

Insoluble fibre – Increases output

Soluble fibre – Slows output

In the table opposite, you can see a list of foods that may thicken or thin stoma output, obstruct the stoma or cause wind. You will find that diet and food tolerances are very individual and these lists are not meant to limit or stop you from eating certain foods, rather to assist you in making informed choices. Some people find that they are able to eat small volumes of the foods without ill effect.

Wind and Odour

Wind (flatus) and odour is caused by the breakdown of food in the bowel and occurs naturally when air is swallowed when breathing or talking. Excess air can also be swallowed by smoking, chewing gum or sucking on hard sweets.

Tips to reduce wind include:

- Eat slowly
- Eat small meals at regular intervals
- Pour fizzy drinks, stir and allow them to settle
- Drink peppermint water, tea or take peppermint capsules
- Eat parsley and yoghurt
- Avoid drinking and eating at the same time
- Avoid talking a lot and eating at the same time
- Avoid drinking through a straw
- Avoid chewing gum
- Reduce insoluble fibre

Tips to reduce odour include:

- Sprays and drops can be used in the stoma appliance
- Change appliance regularly
- Eat parsley and yoghurt
- Avoid foods such as eggs, fish, garlic, beer, strong cheeses and spicy foods
- Reduce insoluble fibre

Dehydration

With a stoma there is a risk of becoming dehydrated as you do not have a colon to reabsorb water and salt. Signs of dehydration include thirst, a dry mouth or dry skin, decreased urine output or dark urine, dizziness, headaches, nausea, achiness and an increased pulse rate.

Tips to avoid dehydration are:

- Try to eat foods that will thicken your output to slow down the amount of fluid you are losing
- You should also add salt to your diet and include salty foods such as bouillon soups, crisps, salty biscuits, pretzels, salted meats, soy sauce and Oxo® cubes
- Include foods and juices that are high in potassium such as bananas, oranges, apricots, tomatoes or grapefruits, squash, potatoes and smooth peanut butter
- If you think you have not drunk enough you should slowly increase your fluid intake. Do not increase it excessively or too quickly. Try filling a bottle of water and sipping throughout the day
- Avoid excessive caffeine as this acts as a diuretic and is found in milk and dark chocolate and cola drinks as well as in tea and coffee
- You may also need fluids which contain salt, such as the World Health Organisation (WHO) solution or the St Mark's Hospital Electrolyte mix solution (E-mix), Dioralyte® rehydration sachets (standard or double strength) and sports drink such as Lucozade®, Powerade® or Gatorade®
- You may require medications that slow down your stoma output such as Loperamide (Immodium®) for a short period. Loperamide must be taken on an empty stomach, at least 30 minutes before meals with a small sip of water

St Mark's Hospital electrolyte mix – this solution lasts 24 hours so you will need to make a new solution daily. The recipe uses the measurements in 5 ml teaspoons:

- 6 level teaspoons of Glucose powder (20 g)
- 1 level teaspoon of Sodium Chloride which is table salt (3.5 g)
- Half a heaped teaspoon of Sodium Bicarbonate also called Bicarbonate of Soda (2.5 g)

Dissolve all ingredients in one litre of water. Some people find that it is better to drink it chilled in the fridge. Do not add ice to it, as this will dilute the solution; however, some people find a splash of cordial or orange squash makes it more palatable. The powdered ingredients can be bought from the chemist or the supermarket.

Changes in colour or consistency

Certain foods or medications may change the colour or consistence of your output from the stoma. This may alarm you but it is worthwhile considering the following:

If you have changes in colour or consistency:

- You may have had a stomach upset or blockage and have not eaten properly for a few hours your output may become green in colour. This is an increase in bile and is perfectly normal
- Your output will return to its normal colour once you have started eating again
- Foods such as beetroot or blackcurrant drinks (Ribena®) may make the output pink or red in colour
- Medication can change the colour of your output: iron and charcoal can make stools black; antacids – white or grey; antibiotics – red, green or grey

If you have not consumed these sorts of food or medications and are still concerned then you should contact a medical professional.

Obstruction

An obstruction can be caused by many factors, one being a food blockage. Symptoms include nausea, abdominal distension or bloating, reduced stoma output, vomiting and abdominal pain. If you experience any of these then it would be advisable to reduce or slow down your eating but keep up your fluid intake. Make sure that you continue to include salt in your oral intake.

Often an obstruction will resolve spontaneously, however, you may find that drinking a glass of water quickly can shift the obstruction. Abdominal massage, exercise (such as walking) or a relaxing bath may help also offer some relief. If you continue to feel unwell, have excruciating pain and vomiting or your stoma has not worked for some time you should consult your GP, pouch nurse or attend your local accident and emergency department. Take note of foods that may have caused your obstruction and avoid them for a few weeks.

Vegetarian or vegan diet

If you have been a vegetarian or a vegan for a long time it is likely that your bowel will be able to tolerate a high fibre diet after surgery but it is still advised to proceed with caution for approximately six weeks. As these diets are based on pulses, legumes and grains which are all fibrous, food from this group must be cooked well or peeled. It may also be wise to shell or blend pulses such as lentils.

Some vegetarians or vegans may lack protein which is vital for wound healing and therefore may be advised on dietary supplementation or alternative sources of protein such as soya, tofu or Asian sea vegetables such as kelp. In some cases you may have to review your lifestyle if complications continue to arise.

Alcohol

Alcohol can be consumed in moderation. Some people may notice a slightly looser bowel motion or an increase in their output the following day. Fizzy drinks such as beer or champagne may produce more wind and you may also have to empty your bag more often.

Medication with a stoma

Medication may still be required even after surgery for a variety of reasons. Some may be used to thicken your stoma output, for pain relief or even to treat inflammation. They may be in tablet or liquid form. It is important that with any medication you read the instructions included within the box.

Medications which can be used to slow down your bowel are:

LOPERAMIDE (also known as Immodium or Norimode®) is a drug that slows down bowel function. It can be bought over the counter or obtained on prescription from your GP. It is recommended that you take these tablets half an hour before meals so that it maximises absorption of your food. You can take 4 mg (2 tablets) four times a day initially and then build this up if the output does not thicken up. The maximum dose that can be taken is up to 16 mg (8 tablets) in a 24 hour period. You may however require higher doses than this but please speak to your pouch nurse or GP before increasing the dose.

CO-PHENOTROPE (Lomotil®) is a combination of 2 drugs and can be used instead of Loperamide.

CODEINE PHOSPHATE is primarily used as an analgesic (painkiller) but one of the side effects is to slow down the bowel. You can take 30–60 mg (1–2 tablets) four times a day with food. This drug can make some people feel quite drowsy so you may prefer to use it at night. Codeine can only be obtained by prescription from your GP.

Medications used to treat inflammation:

STEROIDS (for example Prednisolone) – if you have had surgery due to ulcerative colitis you may still be on steroids even after the operation. It is important that these are not stopped abruptly. The medical team will be able to advise you on what doses you should take daily and how long you should take them for.

PROBIOTICS (for example VSL#3®) can be used as a dietary supplement which may alter the gut flora. This is thought to be useful to prevent a reoccurrence of inflammation.

Medications used for pain relief:

PARACETAMOL can be obtained over the counter and can be quite effective when it builds up in the system.

CODEINE PHOSPHATE is a stronger painkiller. It is primarily used for pain relief but you may find that your stoma output thickens on this painkiller as a side effect of its use.

CODEINE AND PARACETAMOL COMBINATIONS such as co-codamol (Solpadol® and Tylex®) , can be obtained by prescription from your GP.

BUSCOPAN® can be used to help with bowel spasms or windy and cramping pain.

Please note: non-steroidal anti-inflammatory drugs (NSAIDS) such as naproxen, diclofenac (Voltarol®) and ibuprofen (Nurofen®) should be avoided as they can cause ulceration in the small bowel with potential bleeding.

Other medication:

MULTIVITAMINS are optional and are not generally required for patients with a stoma. Most nutritional absorption takes place at the top of your small bowel (near your stomach) not at the end (near your stoma). Some multivitamins may include high levels of iron which in some cases can be an irritant to the bowel causing a higher output from your stoma.

DIORALYTE® is a rehydration drink. This comes in a powder that needs to be mixed with water. It can be bought over the counter and some chemists may have their own brand. Some people find this very handy with a loop stoma to top up their salt and fluid intake. You may need to make it up as double strength, for example, two sachets in 200 ml of water if you are very dehydrated, as a convenient alternative to the St Mark's electrolyte mix.

Lifestyle with a stoma

Following surgery it will take a couple months to recover enough to resume your usual activities and lifestyle. You must remember to listen to your body and reintroduce activities slowly. It is probably better to avoid strenuous household activities such as vacuum cleaning or lawn mowing until you feel able.

It is normal for recovery to take two to three months before confidence with your new stoma is established. Initially having the large bowel removed may mean that the process of digestion does not happen as efficiently, however, over a few months adaptation takes place and the small bowel resumes its role.

You may need to change your diet or lifestyle slightly and keep a check on your fluid and salt levels but overall your quality of life should not be compromised.

Work

Depending on the job you do you may feel able to resume work within a few weeks. Initially it may be wise to accept any offers to work from home or on a part-time basis. You may find it useful to practice the journey into work or your work routine before you return so you can decide how best to fit your stoma into your working day.

You may find it helpful to discuss your condition with the occupational health team or your manager before your return date is set. If you have concerns or feel unable to speak to your employer you could contact your GP, surgeon or pouch nurse for advice.

Returning to education

Most schools or colleges will allow time for recovery but this must be discussed with your Head of School prior to surgery to ensure you will be allowed back on your course. It will also allow you to plan when best to have your operations for example in the school holiday.

If you are struggling to be prepared for examinations you could ask for a letter from your surgeon outlining the surgery as your school may consider exceptions for you or guide you on a more suitable pathway. For younger children a school nurse may be able to assist with initial problems caused by the stoma or offer support if required.

Driving

It is not recommended that you resume driving until you feel comfortable. It is vital that you check your individual policy with your insurance company before attempting to drive, stating that you have had abdominal surgery.

Sport and exercise

Initially light exercise such as walking should be ample to aid your recovery and build up your abdominal strength. Once any wounds have healed you should be able to resume usual exercise and contact sports. It is important you do not strain and breathe correctly. Strenuous activities may cause leakage from the stoma bag and it may be helpful to contact your pouch nurse for advice.

Controlling or disguising smells

We are all much more sensitive to our own smells than other people are and remember that they are unlikely to be as sensitive to it as you. If you are leaking stool and are worried about others noticing an odour:

If you want to control or disguise smells:

- Try to ensure good ventilation of the room you are in
- Use an aromatherapy oil burner, scented candle, joss stick or incense stick, or a dish of pot-pourri
- Use neutralising, deodorant air fresheners which can be purchased from a convenience store, others are available on prescription
- Try striking a match and then blowing it out immediately and allowing the small plume of smoke to drift into the room

Travel

Holidays can be a great incentive to make you feel better but should be planned carefully depending on the mode of travel, availability of

conveniences and duration of your stay. It is advisable to embark on a holiday once you have an established a routine with your stoma and feel confident. It is worth taking extra supplies of stoma bags, your usual medication, anti-diarrhoeal medication and rehydration drinks. Remember a change in diet and lifestyle may affect your stoma and new foods or activities should be undertaken with care. It may be wise to contact your GP, surgeon or pouch nurse for advice prior to embarking on your holiday.

It is highly recommended that you take out a travel insurance policy. Many people with a stoma have been quoted exceptionally high prices but it is worth researching companies tailored to ostomists (people with a stoma) which may offer better deals. It may also be useful to take information with you explaining surgery, your past medical history and other useful contact details. The Ileostomy Association (IA) has a useful travel certificate which can be carried with you and endorsed by your GP (for more information, see the section 'Support Groups').

The European health insurance card

If you plan to travel within the European economic area, a free European health insurance card (EHIC) can be applied for by phone, by post or online.

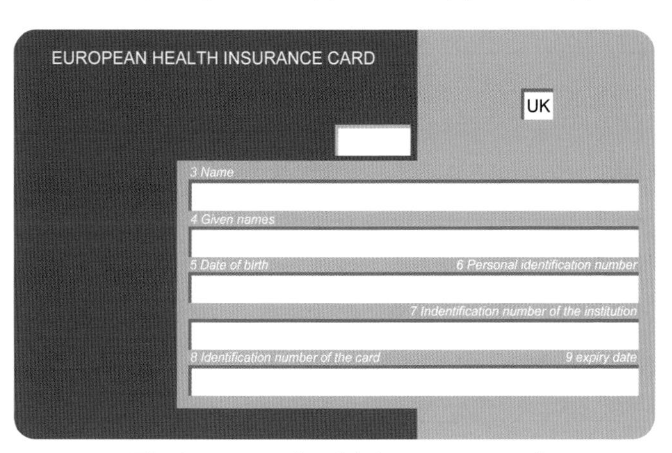

The European health insurance card

Your EHIC lets you get state healthcare at a reduced cost or sometimes for free. It will cover you for treatment of pre-existing medical conditions and any care you need to continue your stay.

RADAR keys offer people access to locked public toilets and can be found in most public places around the country. Official Radar keys cost about five pounds and can be bought from participating local authorities or the Disability Rights UK shop. Some councils and stoma appliance home delivery companies may give them away for free. A National Key Scheme guide is produced for purchase each year, which lists the location of every Radar loo on record. A smartphone app is also available, with added walking and driving directions. Both cost approximately five pounds.

Planning ahead

Being prepared can make living with your stoma easier especially in the early days. Some of these ideas may be helpful if you are uncertain about your stoma function:

Ideas for planning ahead:

- Plan a route with access to public toilets and don't forget your RADAR key
- Take a packet of wet wipes, spare underwear, a new stoma bag and wipes in a small wash bag
- Carry a small squeeze bottle that you can fill with warm water to take into the toilet with you for cleaning
- If you need both hands to get clean, a couple of clothes pegs can keep your clothes from dangling in the wrong place
- A small pocket mirror can be useful to check that you are clean
- Dark colours and pattered fabrics tend to show any stains less than light fabrics so think about your clothing before you go out
- Don't worry too much and relax

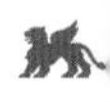

Sex and fertility with a stoma

There is large variation between patients and the effect of surgery on sexual relationships. Some people find that there is little or no effect on their sexual function while others may struggle to come to terms with the effect of a changed body image and managing their new stoma. You may have some degree of pain or discomfort during intercourse after surgery. This problem is usually temporary but for some women pain during intercourse (dyspareunia) can continue after surgery.

Some men may have erectile dysfunction and discomfort but this is also usually temporary. Dyspareunia does improve over time but if you continue to experience problems your surgeon or GP may refer you to an urologist or psychosexual therapist.

Most of the time, your body will let you know when it feels well enough to engage in sexual activity. You may be afraid that your bag will leak or move during sexual activity, experience anxiety about how your partner will react or have negative feelings about yourself and your body image.

If you are not currently in a sexual relationship you may suffer from anxiety about starting a new relationship with someone after undergoing your operation. Patients have reported feeling many of these concerns before and after the surgery, however, many of them can be resolved through discussing these fears. If you would like to discuss any concerns or difficulties you may be experiencing please contact your pouch nurse, surgeon, GP or Support Group (listed at the back of this book).

Do I need to tell my partner about this?

If you are in a sexual relationship we would advise that you talk to your partner as open communication can often resolve the problems. You can be referred for counselling alone or with your partner.

Fertility and pregnancy

Getting pregnant is usually a concern for young couples when there has been a period of ill health followed by the formation of a stoma, however, once the diseased bowel is removed people generally feel more able to plan a family even if they have a stoma. Fertility in young women can be significantly reduced if the rectum is removed, for example in pouch surgery.

Some patients may delay pouch surgery until after they have their family if they are well and it is safe to do so. With the use of laparoscopic surgery and smaller incisions, female fertility may not be as compromised. This is why it is important to discuss all the surgical options with your surgeon or pouch nurse before opting for a pouch.

Once pregnant, patients usually have very little problems with their stoma. As your bump gets bigger the stoma may enlarge or prolapse into the bag. Some patients may report feelings of a blockage or the stoma output slowing down as the bowel may become slightly compressed.

Usually sticking to a light diet or increasing your fluid intake will remedy this problem but in the event of a blockage you are advised to seek medical assistance. It may become difficult to see the stoma when changing the bag and you may need to use a mirror, however, stoma function quickly returns to normal after the birth.

Infertility

Most women may have no problem getting pregnant after surgery. Most couples are advised to have unprotected sex for at least 12 months before seeking assistance. As infertility may be caused by a variety of reasons you are not usually requested to store your eggs or sperm. Egg harvesting and sperm banking is usually performed before radiotherapy or other invasive procedures which may destroy the egg or sperm.

Contraception

Having a stoma does not mean that you do not require contraception. Family planning is an integral part of a sexually active couple. Condoms, diaphragms (caps), implants and three monthly depot injections are frequently used without compromising pouch function. The intrauterine contraceptive device (IUD) or coil is not advised for women who have not had babies, however, some patients with a stoma have used them with no problems. The pill is suitable for most patients, however, if you have had an episode of diarrhoea or vomiting you may need to refrain from sexual activity or add another method of contraception until you feel better. Long-term contraception such as a vasectomy or sterilisation is possible. These should be discussed in depth with your surgeon as some procedures may have to be completed by going back into the abdomen. There are many different methods of contraception available and you should discuss these options with your GP or family planning clinic.

Giving birth

Most women with a stoma will prefer to have a caesarean section (C-section) as they do not wish to risk trauma to the anal sphincter muscles during the birth. Damage to these muscles could mean that you may not be a suitable candidate for pouch surgery. Though you do not have to have a caesarean section it is an option that your obstetrician can discuss with you. There should be no reason why you cannot breast feed, however, you may find you need to increase your oral fluids by drinking more. This may have an influence on your stoma output. If you are concerned about your personal risks contact your pouch nurse or surgeon.

Discharge planning with a stoma

When you are ready for discharge from hospital there are a number of things your pouch nurse will give to you. Below is a checklist.

Please read it and make sure you have everything with you before you leave the hospital.

Discharge checklist:

- Stoma supplies for two weeks
- Contact number for local stoma care nurse if appropriate
- Contact number for St Mark's pouch nurse
- Discharge letter for GP and a copy for yourself
- Outpatient date for stoma review (if you are a local patient)
- Home delivery contact numbers

If you live in Harrow, the pouch nurse will make an appointment to see you in an outpatient clinic until you are well enough to be discharged from follow-up care.

If you are having ongoing problems or wish to discuss any aspects of pouch or stoma care then please ring the pouch care department to speak to the nurse or to make an appointment to attend the pouch care clinic.

Please do not come to the department without making an appointment first as we may be with other patients and unable to see you. If no one is in the office to answer your call please follow the instructions on the answerphone and we will get back to you as soon as possible. This is usually within 24 hours. Please note the phone is not manned on weekends or public holidays and if it is an emergency you are advised to contact your GP, the ward you were discharged from or attend your local emergency department.

If you do not live in the Harrow area, any questions or problems at home are dealt with by your local stoma care nurse. Often things change at home and your local stoma care nurse is the best person to assess these changes. They are based in your area and may visit you at home, which the St Mark's pouch care nurses are unable to do. You can also see your local stoma care nurse as an outpatient in your local hospital and your local stoma care nurse will arrange this with you. The pouch and stoma care nurses are only responsible for the care and management related to your stoma or pouch. If you have a wound that requires dressings then your Practice Nurses will be responsible for this.

The pouch nurses at St Mark's Hospital will speak to anyone contemplating pouch surgery or those who have had pouch surgery even if you are not a patient of the hospital, however, we may be limited in the advice we can offer if you have not been to the hospital before.

Supplies for home use

Before you are discharged from hospital you will need to decide how you will receive your supplies for use at home. You have two options. Both options require a prescription from your GP which you will have to get before supplies are released. Prescription costs can be reduced by obtaining a prescription prepayment certificate (PPC) which is valid for three or twelve months. You are exempt from prescription charges if you have a permanent stoma, are over 60 years of age or exempt by other means such as obtaining relevant benefits. These issues should be discussed with your GP as you will require a medical exemption certificate or PPC.

Option 1: Free delivery of supplies by a home delivery company (HDC)

1. You will go home with two weeks of supplies.
2. The pouch care nurse will ring the HDC and organise a delivery to be sent to your house within two working days.
3. You will need to get a prescription for these supplies from your GP. Your GP will get a letter from the pouch nurse which tells them what products you will need so they can write your prescription.
4. Place the prescription from your GP into the Freepost envelope (which will come with your supplies) and send it to the HDC. Sometimes it may be possible for the HDC to write directly to your GP requesting the prescription. Please ask your pouch care nurse if this is possible and this will be arranged for you.
5. You will receive free wipes and disposal bags with your supplies. If you run out of wipes or disposal bags you can call the HDC and request extra supplies, free of charge.
6. The HDC will contact you in about ten days post-discharge to make sure everything runs smoothly and can answer any questions you have.

7. When you have about two weeks of supplies left, you will need to go to your GP and get a repeat prescription for your stoma products and post it to the HDC. If it has been arranged for the HDC to collect prescriptions on your behalf all you need to do is to call the HDC directly and they will get the prescription from your GP. Continue to do this as long as you have a stoma.

NOTE: If you wish to add to or change your prescription you need to speak to your pouch or stoma nurse first. The HDC is not able to give you alternative products, however, they will let you sample new products for free.

Option 2: Pick up supplies from your chemist

1. You will go home with two weeks of supplies.
2. You will need to get a prescription from your GP and give it to your chemist so they can order the supplies. This may take several days.
3. You then pick up your supplies from the chemist but you may have to return to collect certain items as chemists cannot stock the whole range of stoma products that are available.
4. When you have about two weeks of supplies left you will need to get another prescription from your GP to give to the chemist. Continue to do this for as long as you have a stoma.
5. You will not receive free wipes and disposal bags with your supplies.

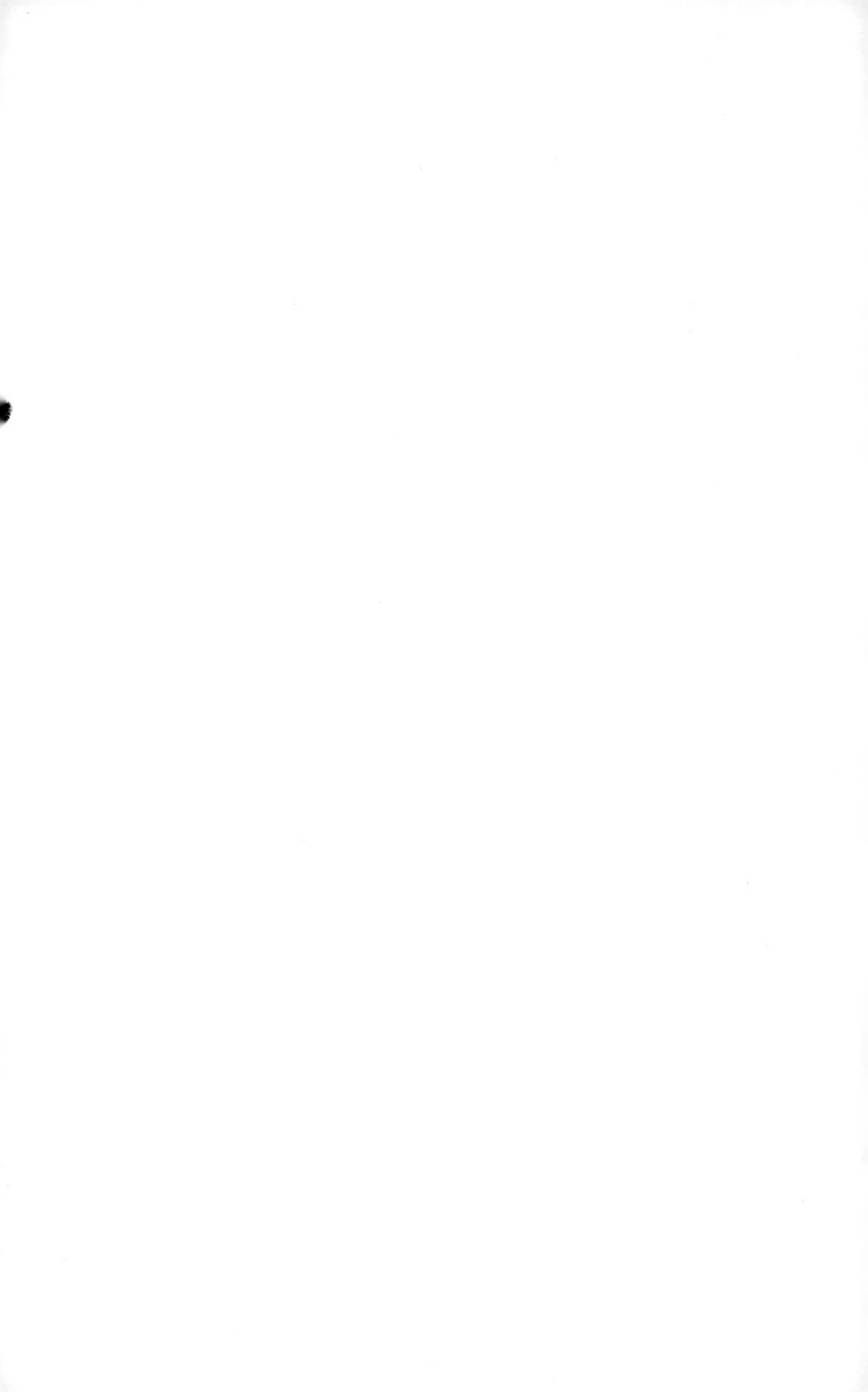

Ileo-anal pouch care

Nurse-led follow-up

As pouch nurses we continue to support you once you have had your stoma closed and your pouch is functioning. Before you leave hospital we will discuss how to 'train' your pouch and show you useful pelvic floor exercises which may also help when emptying the pouch. These methods are sometimes referred to as pouch compliance and urge resistance techniques.

Pouch compliance

It is normal for patients who have undergone two or three stages of surgery to feel a huge sense of relief at having had their stoma closed but this is actually only the beginning of life with a pouch. It can take some time to get used to the pouch and how it functions, anything from 6–24 months. The key point to make is that you need to be patient as function can be quite unsettled for the first few weeks as you gradually introduce new foods into your diet. Pouches like routine so it is important that you eat little and often, listen to what your pouch is telling you with regard to emptying and try not to get too anxious. Stress can have a big impact on bowel function, and pouches in particular, so if your pouch function deteriorates consider whether your routine and stress levels have changed.

Urge resistance

Having had ulcerative colitis it is likely that you will have experienced urgency when having a flare-up of the disease and also potentially incontinence. Your brain will be tuned into telling you that if you get the sensation of needing to go to the toilet you need to go urgently. You need to override your brain telling you this and gradually build up your urge resistance as with the pouch you should not have urgency. In the initial days following closure of your stoma you will have the sensation of needing to empty your pouch but you should wait a few minutes before going to the toilet, thereby overriding your brain and training your pouch. Day by day you can build up your urge resistance or how long you hold on for to a time that is acceptable for you. If you delay evacuation for too long you can get a build-up of wind which can be uncomfortable, though you will soon be able to establish what suits you best. In the time that you had your loop stoma, your pouch would have been producing mucus so it may be that you have built up a degree of urge resistance already.

Pelvic floor exercises

The pelvic floor muscle runs along the bottom of the pelvis and encompasses the rectum and anus. Exercises can be done to improve the strength of the pelvic floor but this need to be done routinely in order for them to be effective. Strengthening the pelvic floor can sometimes help if you are experiencing leakage from the pouch.

With women it is advised that the anus and vagina are squeezed as tightly as possible and you imagine you are picking up two coins, one with the anus and one with the vagina. This position should be held for five seconds, relaxed for ten seconds and then repeated. With men the anus should be squeezed, held for five seconds, relaxed for ten seconds and then repeated. If men are sitting down and their testicles are lifting off the chair then they are using the right technique. The buttocks should not be squeezed as this does not help the pelvic floor. One way of avoiding squeezing the buttocks is to stand up and point your toes inwards as if you are standing pigeon-toed. If possible you should try and do five of the exercises in a row five times a day and incorporate them into your daily activities. You can do the exercises sitting, standing or lying down so you could try doing them whilst brushing your teeth, on the phone or waiting at traffic lights.

Out-patient support

The support from the pouch nurses will continue even if you have been discharged from the care of the doctors. You have access to our telephone advice line and we can also be contacted by e-mail and aim to reply to these as soon as we can. Sometimes we prefer to speak to you over the phone so we can clarify things or obtain a full history of your concerns in order to help you. We can offer advice with regard to pouch function, diet or lifestyle and with the information you provide, may be able to diagnose problems over the phone. If deemed necessary we can liaise with your GP regarding prescriptions and organise investigations and clinic appointments.

You may be reviewed in the surgical clinic a few weeks after you have had your stoma closed, however more commonly you will see the pouch nurse three or four times during the first year after the stoma is closed to help you adjust to your pouch. Depending on your health you will then be discharged back to your GP, however, if you have a history of primary sclerosing cholangitis (a liver condition), dysplasia (precancerous cell changes) or a cancer when your large bowel was removed or a history of chronic pouchitis (inflammation in the pouch) then you will not be discharged from follow-up at St Mark's Hospital.

We also run rapid access nurse-led clinics if you need to be seen for assessment and do not require a doctor. You can easily book into these by contacting the pouch nurse telephone advice line. If you have been discharged and need to come back to clinic to see either a pouch nurse or doctor then you will require a referral from your GP. The referral letter can be faxed directly to us so an appointment can be made for you more quickly.

It is recommended that all patients with a pouch have annual blood tests done by their GP once they are discharged. These should include full blood count, urea and electrolytes, liver function tests, calcium, ferritin, folate, vitamin B12 and vitamin D. Vitamin B12 is absorbed at the end of your small bowel (unlike other vitamins which are absorbed at the top). Though most patients have a store of vitamin B12 it may need to be replaced in the future with an injection every few months. You will need to remind your GP to check your bloods, as it is not routinely offered.

Lifestyle with a pouch

Following surgery it will take a couple months to recover enough to resume your usual activities and lifestyle. You must remember to listen to your body and reintroduce activities slowly. It is probably better to avoid strenuous household activities such as vacuum cleaning or lawn mowing until you feel able.

It is normal for recovery to take six months to two years following pouch surgery before confidence with your new pouch is established as the pouch has to settle down into its new role. Initially having the large bowel and rectum removed may mean that the process of digestion does not happen as efficiently, however, over a few months adaptation takes place and the small bowel resumes its role.

You may need to change your diet or lifestyle slightly and keep a check on your iron and salt levels but overall your quality of life should not be compromised.

Work

Depending on the job you do you may feel able to resume work within a few weeks. Initially it may be wise to accept any offers to work from home or on a part-time basis.

You may find it useful to practice the journey into work or your work routine before you return so you can decide how best to fit your pouch into your working day. You may find it helpful to discuss your condition with the occupational health team or your manager before your return date is set.

If you have concerns or feel unable to speak to your employer you could contact your GP, surgeon or pouch nurse for advice.

Returning to education

Most schools or colleges will allow time for recovery but this must be discussed with your Head of School prior to surgery to ensure you will be allowed back on your course. It will also allow you to plan when best to have your operations for example in the school holiday.

If you are struggling to be prepared for examinations you could ask for a letter from your surgeon outlining the surgery so your school may consider exceptions for you or guide you on a more suitable pathway. For younger children a school nurse may be able to assist with initial problems caused by the pouch or offer support if required.

Driving

It is not recommended that you resume driving until you feel comfortable. It is vital that you check your individual policy with your insurance company before attempting to drive stating that you have had abdominal surgery.

Sport and exercise

Initially light exercise such as walking should be ample to aid your recovery and build up your abdominal strength. Once any wounds have healed you should be able to resume usual exercise and contact sports. It is important you do not strain and breathe correctly. Strenuous activities may cause leakage from the pouch and it may be helpful to wear a pad. For individual advice you should contact your GP, surgeon or pouch nurse for advice.

Controlling or disguising smells

We are all much more sensitive to our own smells than other people are but remember that they are unlikely to be as sensitive to it as you. If you are leaking stool and are worried about others noticing an odour you may feel more comfortable wearing a small sanitary pad.

If you want to control or disguise smells:

- Try to ensure good ventilation of the room you are in
- Use an aromatherapy oil burner, scented candle, joss stick or incense stick, or a dish of pot-pourri
- When emptying your pouch use a neutralising, deodorant air freshener which can be purchased from a convenience store
- Others are available on prescription

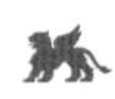

Travel

Holidays can be a great incentive to make you feel better but should be planned carefully depending on the mode of travel, availability of conveniences and duration of your stay. It is advisable to embark on a holiday once you have an established a routine with your pouch and feel confident.

It is worth taking extra supplies of barrier creams, your usual medication, anti-diarrhoeal medication, rehydration drinks and antibiotics if you need them or are prone to pouchitis. Remember a change in diet and lifestyle may affect your pouch function and new foods or activities should be undertaken with care.

It may be wise to contact your GP, surgeon or pouch nurse for advice prior to embarking on your holiday.

It is highly recommended that you take out a travel insurance policy. Many people with a pouch have been quoted exceptionally high prices but it is worth researching companies tailored to ostomists (people with a stoma) which may offer better deals, even for pouch patients.

It may also be useful to take information with you explaining pouch surgery, your past medical history and other useful contact details. The Ileostomy Association (IA) has a useful travel certificate which can be carried with you and endorsed by your GP (see details under support groups).

If you plan to travel within the European economic area a free European health insurance card (EHIC) can be applied for by phone, by post or online.

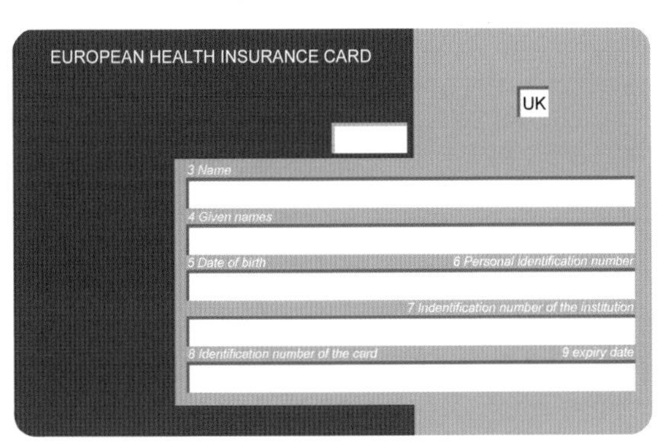

The European health insurance card

Your EHIC lets you get state health care at a reduced cost or sometimes for free. It will cover you for treatment of pre-existing medical conditions and any care you need to continue your stay.

RADAR keys offer people access to locked public toilets and can be found in most public places around the country. Official Radar keys cost about five pounds and can be bought from participating local authorities or the Disability Rights UK shop. Some councils and stoma appliance home delivery companies may give them away for free. A 'National Key Scheme' guide is produced for purchase each year, which lists the location of every Radar loo on record. A smartphone app is also available, with added walking and driving directions. Both are currently five pounds.

Planning ahead

Being prepared can make living with your pouch easier especially in the early days. Some of these ideas may be helpful if you are uncertain about your pouch function:

Ideas for planning ahead:

- Plan a route with access to public toilets (don't forget your RADAR key)
- Take a packet of wet wipes, barrier creams, spare underwear and an extra pad in a small wash bag
- Carry a small squeeze bottle that you can fill with warm water to take into the toilet with you for cleaning
- If you need both hands to get clean or change a pad, a couple of clothes pegs can keep your clothes from dangling in the wrong place
- A small pocket mirror can be useful to check that you are clean
- Dark colours and pattered fabrics tend to show any stains less than light fabrics so think about your clothing before you go out
- Don't worry too much and relax

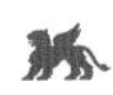

Sex and fertility with a pouch

There is a large variation between patients and the effect of pouch surgery on sexual relationships. Some people find that there is little or no effect on their sexual function while others may struggle to come to terms with the effect of a changed body image and managing their new pouch. You may have some degree of pain or discomfort during intercourse after surgery. This problem is usually temporary but for some women pain during intercourse (dyspareunia) can continue after surgery.

Some men may have erectile dysfunction and discomfort but this is also usually temporary. Dyspareunia does improve over time but if you continue to experience problems your surgeon or GP could refer you to an urologist or psychosexual therapist. Most of the time your body will let you know when it feels well enough to engage in sexual activity. You may be afraid that you will be incontinent during sexual activity, experience anxiety about how your partner will react or have negative feelings about yourself and your body image.

If you are not currently in a sexual relationship you may suffer from anxiety about starting a new relationship with someone after undergoing your operation. Patients have reported feeling many of these concerns before and after the pouch surgery, however, many of them can be resolved through discussing these fears. If you would like to discuss any concerns or difficulties you may be experiencing please contact your pouch nurse, surgeon, GP or support group (listed at the back of this book). If you are in a sexual relationship we would advise that you talk to your partner as open communication can often resolve the problems. You can be referred for counselling alone or with your partner.

Fertility and pregnancy

Getting pregnant is usually a concern for young couples when there has been a period of ill health followed by a series of surgical interventions.

Females: Fertility in young women can be significantly reduced if the rectum is removed, for example in pouch surgery. Some patients may delay pouch surgery until after they have their family if they are well and it is safe to do so.

One of the advantages of laparoscopic surgery is that the amount of adhesions around the ovary and tubes is so reduced that it may increase the chances of achieving pregnancy. As we now use laparoscopic surgery more frequently for pouch surgery it appears that this may certainly play a part in increasing the chances of achieving pregnancy. This is why it is important to discuss all the surgical options with your surgeon or pouch nurse.

Males: The nerves that control ejaculation and erection are very close to the rectum. These nerves can be damaged when the rectum is being removed. The risk of nerve damage at this type of surgery is about 3% in experienced hands and is thought to be reduced by laparoscopic surgery as there is a better view of the nerves at surgery.

In some situations the effects of nerve injury are not permanent and function can return within a few months after surgery. The effects of this complication can manifest in two ways; lack of erection or retrograde ejaculation. Lack of erection can be partial or full and in most situations appear to respond to medications such as Viagra®. Retrograde ejaculation is when the sperm enters the bladder rather than coming out through the penis. This has effects on the fertility of a male and may require a comprehensive discussion with your surgeon.

Once pregnant, people usually have very little problem with their pouch. As the baby gets bigger though some people may experience frequency or urgency getting to the toilet, especially in the last trimester. Some patients may have some degree of leakage from the pouch and are advised to wear a small pad, however, pouch function quickly returns to normal after the birth.

Infertility

Some women may have difficulty getting pregnant after pouch surgery. Most couples are advised to have unprotected sex for at least twelve months before seeking assistance. Most investigations will be done under your local obstetric team who may sometimes seek advice from your surgeon.

Some women may qualify for one round of in vitro fertilisation (IVF) on the NHS after pouch surgery. It is worthwhile to discuss all your options with your surgeon or pouch nurse. As infertility may be caused by a variety of reasons you are not usually requested to store your eggs or sperm. Egg harvesting and sperm banking is usually performed before radiotherapy or other invasive procedures which may destroy the egg or sperm.

 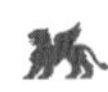

Contraception

Having a pouch does not mean that you do not require contraception. Family planning is an integral part of a sexually active couple. Condoms, diaphragms (caps), implants and three monthly depot injections are frequently used without compromising pouch function.

The intrauterine contraceptive device (IUD) or coil is not advised for women who have not had babies. Patients with a pouch have used an IUD successfully when their family is complete. The pill is suitable for most patients, however, if you have had an episode of diarrhoea or vomiting you may need to refrain from sexual activity or add another method of contraception until you feel better.

Long-term contraception such as a vasectomy or sterilisation is possible. These should be discussed in-depth with your surgeon as some procedures may have to be completed by going back into the abdomen. There are many different methods of contraception available and you should discuss these options with your GP or family planning clinic.

Giving birth

Most women with a pouch will prefer to have a caesarean section (C-section) as they do not wish to risk trauma to their anal sphincter muscles during the birth. Damage to these muscles could mean that the ability to hold their pouch contents can be reduced. Though you do not have to have a caesarean section it is an option that your obstetrician can discuss with you.

There should be no reason why you cannot breast feed, however, you may find you need to increase your oral fluids by drinking more. This may have an influence on your pouch output. If you are concerned about your personal risks contact your pouch nurse or surgeon.

Smear tests

After pouch surgery it is still important you continue to have your required smear tests. Some women may find it more uncomfortable when the speculum is inserted into the vagina. Sometimes it may be a struggle to insert the speculum or to see the cervix. This can happen even to women who have not had a pouch. It is best to try and relax as much as possible or change position slightly. Having a routine smear test should not interfere with your pouch or pouch function.

Menstrual cycle and the menopause

Most women may notice a change in their pouch function around the time of their menstrual cycle. This can involve a more liquid stool, frequent or urgent emptying of the pouch or associated pelvic pain and discomfort. This change in pouch function can be prolonged in older women during menopause.

The main cause is due to the fluctuation of hormones which pass through the small bowel. Hormonal changes may be surgically induced by pelvic surgery perhaps because of a compromised blood supply to the ovaries. Most women find that pouch function returns to normal after the menstrual period or the menopause.

Pouch diet

Dietary requirements will vary from one person to another and will depend on your individual lifestyle and eating patterns. These recommendations serve only as a guide and must be tailored to individual need.

Though your body is adapting to living without a colon you will still lose fluid and some salt through your pouch so it is important that dietary precautions are taken in the first few weeks after stoma reversal surgery. You will also need to drink approximately 1.5–2 litres (8–10 glasses) of fluid a day to make up for the fluid loss and to avoid becoming dehydrated. It is essential that you continue to include salt in your diet. This means cooking with salt, adding salt to your food or eating foods and snacks that contain salt. You need about a teaspoon of salt per day after stoma reversal surgery. If you have been advised to avoid salt for a medical reason such as high blood pressure you may wish to discuss this further with your pouch nurse, GP or surgeon as it is likely you will still need to increase your salt intake to prevent dehydration.

After surgery you will be allowed to eat a light, low residue diet as soon as you are able to, which can be the same day as the operation. It is important to have a balanced diet in order to promote healing and prevent infections. Dietary restrictions occur with a new pouch (for approximately four weeks after stoma reversal) as the join in the bowel where the stoma has been closed will still be swollen. After four weeks you can reintroduce most foods. Your dietary requirements will differ according to your personal situation and lifestyle, however, once your pouch is established you may begin to enjoy foods you probably avoided with your stoma, however, it may take 6–24 months before your pouch is fully established and you feel confident enough to know which foods and in which volumes are suitable for your lifestyle.

New pouch (first four weeks after stoma closure)

In the first four weeks after your stoma is closed and your pouch starts working your diet will be similar to when you first had a stoma. Initially some adjustments may be required to your diet to prevent obstruction, excessive odour, wind or a high output.

Most people with a new pouch will not be able to pass wind without sitting on the toilet. You may find it easier to eat small frequent meals and snacks rather than three full meals a day.

It is advisable to eat a low residue diet which avoids insoluble fibre. The aim of this diet is to prolong the intestinal transit time of the stool thereby decreasing the frequency of evacuating your pouch. Over time (12–18 months) the bacteria will colonise the pouch and adaptive changes will occur that assist the pouch to work more effectively. Once these adaptive changes have taken place most people find they can eat a much more varied diet including insoluble fibre.

Please remind yourself about preventing dehydration, wind and odour and alcohol intake by revisiting the diet section as the diet post stoma reversal is basically the same as a new stoma diet.

Anal irritation

Some foods can cause anal irritation. These include spicy foods, nuts, citrus fruits and juices, raw fruit and vegetables, dried fruits (such as raisins or dates), popcorn and coconut. These foods should be reintroduced slowly.

Obstruction

An obstruction with a pouch can be caused by many factors, one being a food blockage. Symptoms include nausea, abdominal distension or bloating, reduced pouch output, vomiting or abdominal pain. If you experience any of these then it would be advisable to reduce or slow down your eating but keep up your fluid intake. Make sure that you continue to include salt in your oral intake. Often an obstruction will resolve spontaneously, however, you may find that drinking a glass of water quickly can shift the obstruction. Abdominal massage, exercise (such as walking) or a relaxing bath may help also offer some relief.

If you continue to feel unwell, have excruciating pain and vomiting or your pouch has not worked for some time you should consult your GP, pouch nurse or attend your local accident and emergency department. If you are admitted into hospital it is usually for a 'watch and wait' approach. This is where you are rehydrated with an intravenous infusion, given pain relief and antiemetic medication to stop you being sick. An X-ray of your abdomen and pelvis may be taken. Take note of foods that may have caused your obstruction and avoid these for a few weeks. Reintroduce them with caution.

Remember, an operation is not the first line treatment for an obstruction.

Anal skin care

Skin is made up of layers of tissue which protect your body. Injury can peel these layers apart causing redness and pain or even cause blisters and bulky eruptions. When you eat, the food is mixed with digestive juices (acids and enzymes) which liquidise your food so that the nutrients can be absorbed by the small intestine. Normally, this would then be passed into the large intestine to absorb the water and produce formed stool. In your operation your large bowel was removed which is the reason your pouch output is more fluid. Your stool still contains digestive acids and enzymes which can easily damage the skin on your bottom.

Now your stoma has been closed it is likely that you may get a sore bottom from time to time. If you find that your pouch output is high (ten times or more in 24 hours) sore skin is inevitable as your bottom is not ideally suited to this new situation. This is usually caused by bowel motions being in contact with the pouch-anal anastomosis (the join from your pouch to the anus) or leakage of stool from the pouch into the anal canal. This can be in association with an itch and/or anal burning. Taking good care of the skin around the anus can help stop these problems occurring. Barrier creams, barrier wipes, haemorrhoid preparations such as Anusol® or high strength (over 70%) aloe vera gels have been noted to be helpful.

Hints and tips to avoid anal soreness and itching

To avoid anal soreness and itching, consider the following:

- Keep the area clean by washing and drying after every motion
- Apply cream or barrier wipe after every motion. Use a mirror to assist cleaning and applying barrier creams
- Avoid excessive use of creams and make sure these are completely washed away before reapplication
- Have regular baths or use a bidet
- Portable bidets are available from the chemist, however, many people sit over a bathtub and use a shower head as a makeshift bidet
- Use moist toilet paper or wipes
- Avoid rubbing, perfumed talc or soap
- Keep the anal area dry
- Wear loose cotton underwear and avoid tight fitting trousers
- Consider thickening the bowel output by use of drugs such as Loperamide or Codeine Phosphate
- Some foods can increase itching or burning, examples of which are coconut and citrus fruit

Suggested skin protectors on prescription

- Ostoguard® Barrier Cream with aloe vera and lavender, product code: RMC2
- Coloplast Brava® Barrier Cream 60 ml tube, product code: 12000
- Simcare Chiron Barrier Cream 52 g tube, product code: WM 102-01-A
- 3M Cavilon™ Durable Barrier Cream 92 g tube, product code: 3392E
- Clinimed® LBF (Liquid Barrier Film) wipes, product code: 3820
- Opus Healthcare Skin Safe skin wipes, product code: 6600
- Pelican Ultra Barrier Cream, product code: 130105
- LaVera Barrier Cream, product code: 3301

Suggested skin protectors available from the chemist

- Sudocrem®
- Vasoline® / Vaseline®
- Metanium® nappy rash ointment
- Anusol® cream or suppository
- Moist wipes

There are a number of other conditions that could give you discomfort or pain in your anal area. We try to avoid surgical intervention as much as possible as we do not want to cause damage or trauma to the anal sphincter muscles or the pouch itself. Most of the time your surgeon, pouch nurse or GP can advise you on what to do.

Haemorrhoids may have developed prior to your pouch being formed or they may develop once you have had your pouch for a period of time. These are small vessels within the inside lining of the anus. These can sometimes become engorged with blood and swell causing bleeding or discomfort. The discomfort can sometimes be relieved by applying a cream or suppository. These can be bought from your local pharmacy.

Fissures are small tears in the lining of the anus and can be extremely painful. It will often be necessary for a pouch nurse or doctor to examine the pouch using an instrument called a proctoscope to look at the inside of the anal canal or pouch for evidence of fissures. The best treatment for a fissure is to apply a small amount of cream to the area. It will sting as it is an open wound but this will settle and it will help protect the area. The two creams commonly used are Diltiazem cream and Glyceryl Trinitrate ointment (GTN) which are available on prescription.

Anal skin tags are an excess growth of skin in the anal region. They are completely harmless but can cause pain and itching as they make cleaning the anus difficult. If the skin tags are problematic they can be removed by a surgeon.

Medication with a pouch

Medication may still be required even after pouch surgery for a variety of reasons. Some may be used to thicken your pouch output, for pain relief or even to treat inflammation. They may be in tablet or liquid form or administered into your pouch as an enema or suppository. It is important that with any medication you read the instructions included within the box. Most pouch patients may need different doses and this will be discussed with you before start taking any medication.

Medications used to slow down your bowel

Loperamide (also known as Immodium® or Norimode®) is a drug that slows the function of the bowel down. It can be bought over the counter or obtained on prescription from your GP. You can take 2 mg (one tablet) four times a day initially and then build this up if the output does not thicken up. It is recommended that you take these tablets half an hour before meals to maximise absorption of your food. The maximum dose recommended is 16 mg (eight tablets), however, you may require higher doses than this but please speak to your pouch nurse or GP before increasing your dose.

Co-phenotrope (Lomotil®) is a combination of two drugs and can be used instead of Loperamide.

Codeine Phosphate is primarily used as an analgesic (painkiller) but one of the side effects is to slow down the bowel. You can take 30–60 mg four times a day with food. This drug can make some people feel drowsy so you may prefer to use it at night. Codeine can only be obtained by prescription from your GP.

Amitriptyline is an anti-depressant, however, in very low doses it is helpful in reducing the pouch frequency if this is caused by an over sensitive pouch. Amitriptyline is also used to help with nerve pain especially in the anus.

Ispaghula Husk (Fybogel™) is a bulk-forming laxative that increases the faecal mass and may be used to slow down your pouch function as it absorbs excess fluid. Psyllium Husk is a powder or capsule which also adds fibre in the diet causing more fluid to be absorbed in your small bowel, however, extra fibre supplements can cause excess wind and cramping pains.

Medications used to treat inflammation

Steroids may be used to treat pouchitis if antibiotics are not effective, however, this is not common practice and needs to be discussed with your medical team.

Antibiotics are the main treatment option and are commonly prescribed for pouchitis. Some patients may have a two or four week course of antibiotics whilst others may rely on extended doses to control their pouchitis. Occasionally you may be asked to give a stool sample which is screened for other infections and to determine what types of bacteria reside in your pouch. We can then decide which antibiotic should be most effective. This will be discussed and agreed by your surgeon, pouch nurse and GP.

Ciprofloxacin is the most frequently used antibiotic in the treatment of pouchitis with the least side effects. Long-term use of ciprofloxacin may result in tendon damage.

Metronidazole is often taken in combination with ciprofloxacin. You must not drink alcohol when taking it. Side effects can include gastrointestinal disturbances including nausea and vomiting, furred coating on the tongue, change in taste, sore mouth and lack of appetite. Sometimes patients who are on this drug for a long time may develop numbness in their fingers.

Augmentin™ is also known as Co-amoxiclav. There are minimal common side effects with this drug, however, is not advised if you are allergic to penicillin.

Trimethoprim is usually used for bladder infections but can be used for pouchitis after stool screening. Side effects can include nausea and vomiting and skin conditions.

Nitrofurantoin Side effects can include loss of appetite, nausea and vomiting and diarrhoea. Long term use can potentially cause harm to the kidneys and liver and your GP may need to check these with blood tests from time to time.

Colistin is used less commonly in the treatment of pouchitis.

Probiotics for example VSL#3® can be used as a dietary supplement which will alter the gut flora. This is thought to be useful to prevent a reoccurrence of pouchitis once antibiotic treatment has been effective but you may incur other costs to obtain it.

Medication used for treatment of the cuff

- **Mesalazine suppositories** (also known as Asacol®, Pentasa® or Salofalk®)
- **Prednisolone suppositories**
- **Predfoam® enemas**

These can be self-administered into the pouch. They are either in the form of suppositories or enemas and aim to treat the inflammation in the cuff. Suppositories tend to work better as they stay longer in the pouch than an enema and should be administered at a time when the pouch is less likely to open (for example, at night).

Medications used for the treatment of fissures in the anal canal

- **Glyceryl Trinitrate 0.2%** (or 0.4% ointment available at the chemist)
- **Diltiazem 2% cream** (only obtainable from the hospital pharmacy)

In order to help heal the fissure it will be necessary to apply a cream or ointment directly to the affected area. This will increase the blood flow to the anus and help healing. You must obtain medical advice before starting treatment as the side effects can include headaches, dizziness, localised bleeding or itching.

Medications used for pain relief

- **Paracetamol** can be obtained over the counter and can be quite effective when it builds up in the system.
- **Codeine Phosphate** is a stronger painkiller. It is primarily used for pain relief but you may find that your pouch output thickens on this painkiller as a side effect of its use.
- **Codeine and Paracetamol combinations** such as co-codamol (Solpadol® and Tylex®) can be obtained by prescription from your GP.
- **Buscopan®** can be used to help with bowel spasms or windy and cramping pain.

 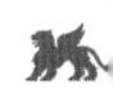

NOTE: Non-steroidal anti-inflammatory drugs (NSAIDS) such as Diclofenac (Voltarol®) and Ibuprofen (Nurofen®) should be avoided as they can cause ulceration in the pouch with potential bleeding.

Medications used to aid the insertion of Medena™ catheters or Hegar dilators into the pouch

- **Lidocaine gel** will lubricate and numb the anal area as it has a local anaesthetic in it. Unfortunately it is only available in 100 g pots via Northwick Park and St Mark's Hospital pharmacy. You could ask your GP for a prescription which can be taken to your chemist. Your chemist can then create an account for you to get Lidocaine gel locally. The number for the pharmacy at Northwick Park and St Mark's Hospital is 0208 869 2295.
- **Instillagel®** is a similar product to Lidocaine but is not as thick in consistency and contains chlorhexidine. These come in pre-filled syringes and can be obtained on prescription.
- **KY-Jelly®** is a water-based gel without local anaesthetic.

Rehydration fluids

ST MARK'S HOSPITAL ELECTROLYTE MIX is an alternative rehydration drink and can be made up at home. The solution lasts 24 hours so you will need to make a new solution daily if required. The recipe uses the measurements in 5 ml teaspoons:

- Six level teaspoons of glucose powder (20 g)
- One level teaspoon of Sodium Chloride which is table salt (3.5 g)
- Half a heaped teaspoon of Sodium Bicarbonate also called Bicarbonate of Soda (2.5 g)

Dissolve all ingredients in one litre of water. Some people find that it is better to drink if chilled in the fridge. Do not add ice to it as this will dilute the solution. Some people find a splash of cordial or orange squash makes it more palatable. The powdered ingredients can be bought from the chemist or the supermarket.

- **Dioralyte®** is a rehydration drink. This comes in a powder that needs to be mixed with water. It can be bought over the counter and some chemists may have their own brand. Some people find this very handy to top up their salt and fluid intake. If you become very dehydrated you may need 'double strength' Dioralyte which is two sachets instead of one, in the recommended amount of water therefore it is recommended that you mix ten sachets of Dioralyte in one litre of water and sip over 24 hours.
- **Isotonic drinks** replace fluids and electrolytes that are lost if you have frequent pouch motions or do exercise. Drinks such as Lucozade™, Powerade™ and Gatorade™ are readily available from supermarkets or convenience stores and are handy to carry with you.

Other medication

Multivitamins are optional and are not generally required for patients with a pouch. Most nutritional absorption takes place at the top of your small bowel (near your stomach) not at the end (in your pouch). Some multivitamins may include high levels of iron which in some cases can be an irritant to the bowel causing a higher output from your pouch.

Please seek advice from your surgeon, pouch nurse or GP if you have any concerns or questions regarding these medications.

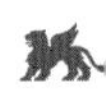

Pouch complications

Complications can occur at any time after the stoma is closed. The two main complications include obstruction and infection. It is important that you seek professional medical advice if you are concerned so that the appropriate investigations into diagnosing and treating the problem can commence.

Leak/infection

Patients always undergo a pouchogram to check that there is no leak from the pouch before the stoma is closed. Stoma closure is a relatively minor procedure. A cut is made around the stoma itself, the bowel is then closed by stitches and then the hole in the abdomen is also closed. Only rarely is it necessary to open the abdomen more extensively. Very occasionally the joins in the bowel may leak. This can lead to an infection and may require further surgery. Symptoms can include anal or abdominal pain, excessive mucus discharge from the pouch, back pain, a fever and generally feeling unwell. If there has been a leak it can sometimes take a while for symptoms to materialise, however, if you are concerned you must seek medical advice.

Pelvic collection

A pelvic collection (sepsis) occurs when there is a leak at the join where the pouch is attached to the anus or any point along the joins created to make the pouch. It is often an early complication of pouch creation but very occasionally can manifest later. The treatment for this is to drain the collection in the pelvis which most often can be done by CT or ultrasound guidance. Sometimes surgery to drain this is required. It may take quite a while to heal the area that is leading to the sepsis and in the case of sepsis, the closure of the stoma can be delayed. In rare circumstances a permanent stoma, recreation of the pouch or removal of the pouch may be required.

Wound infection

Dressings are usually recommended on the wound following stoma closure and will be monitored by the district/practice nurse once discharged. Many surgeons prefer to leave the stoma closure site slightly open to allow the wound to heal completely from the bottom upwards. If you are worried that any of your wounds or ports sites become more painful, red, hardened or oozing fluid please seek medical advice.

Ileus

Food passes through the bowel with a regular contraction and relaxation of the muscles known as peristalsis. Initially in hospital, when the stoma is closed sometimes peristalsis slows down and this causes gastrointestinal fluids and food to stop moving through the bowel. This can lead to symptoms of a blockage in which the abdomen becomes bloated, painful and you may feel nauseous. The pouch can also sometimes stop working as nothing is able to pass through. If you begin to vomit then it is commonly advised that you stop eating and a nasogastric tube is inserted in order to relieve the pressure on the abdomen. A member of nursing staff will insert a thin plastic tube up through the nose, down the back of the throat and into the stomach. The tube would be secured to the nose with a piece of tape and then a drainage bag attached to the other end. This enables the stomach contents to drain into the bag and relieve some of the bloated feeling and nausea. Intravenous fluids would also be needed during this period in order to keep you hydrated and until you are able to eat again.

Blockage

A partial blockage may occur any time after surgery and usually this is caused by a food bolus (undigested food) stopping the natural movement in the pouch. Sometimes the bowel may twist slightly (volvulus) causing the symptoms of a blockage (see above). It is advised that you stop eating and drink fluids only for a few hours to attempt to 'flush' the obstruction through. It may be wise to drink a couple glasses of water quickly to help move things along. Some people find a brisk walk, abdominal massage or relaxing in a warm bath may help restart the pouch, however, if you do become more bloated, the pain increases or you begin to vomit, you must seek medical advice immediately!

If you are admitted into hospital it is usually for a 'watch and wait' approach. You will be rehydrated with an intravenous infusion, given pain relief or antiemetic medication to stop you being sick. Sometimes a nasogastric tube will be inserted into your nose to allow the pouch to decompress. You may be sent for an X-ray of your abdomen and pelvis to determine the cause of the blockage. The bowel usually starts functioning again on its own without the need for surgery but it can sometimes take a few days for everything to settle. If surgery is required this will immediately relieve the blockage, but remember, **an operation is not the first line of treatment for an obstruction!**

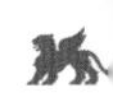

Incomplete emptying

Sometimes you may find you are not able to empty your pouch effectively and it is not due to undigested food. This may occur on a few separate occasions or become a long-standing problem. Difficulty emptying can also be caused by:

- Ineffective emptying techniques
- Stricture (narrowing) within the pouch or at the join between the pouch and the anus
- Retained rectum which was not removed in your previous operation
- Inflammation (for example, pouchitis)
- Functional problems in which the cause is not clear

In order to help empty your pouch it may be useful to position yourself a certain way on the toilet. Some patients find that they will need to stand up halfway through emptying the pouch, in order to allow the stool to flow easier. Some patients massage their abdomen and try breathing exercises to relax. It is important that you do not strain. The correct position for emptying your bowels is illustrated in these pages. If positioning does not help with the emptying of your pouch it may be necessary to learn how to use a plastic tube known as a Medena™ catheter. This helps drain the faeces from the pouch. The pouch nurse will be able to teach you how to do this either in a clinic or on the ward.

Instructions for using a Medena™ catheter

The equipment you will need is as follows: a Medena™ catheter, lubricating jelly or Lidocaine gel, a 50 ml bladder syringe, 50 ml of warm tap water. Then:

- Fill the syringe with the tap water
- Lubricate the end of the catheter and eyelets with jelly or gel and if preferred apply some to the anal area
- Hold the catheter between the thumb and forefinger, approximately 3–4 inches from the eyelets
- Insert the catheter into the anus stooping or sitting on the toilet, depending on which is more comfortable. Stop when your fingers reach the buttocks
- Check the other end of the catheter is aimed towards the toilet bowl
- When the Medena™ catheter is in the correct position, flatus or faecal fluid will be passed

̶Correct position for opening your bowels

Step one

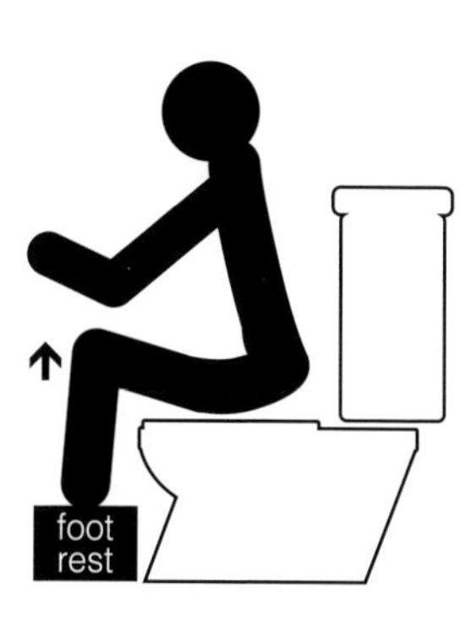

Knees higher than hips

Step two

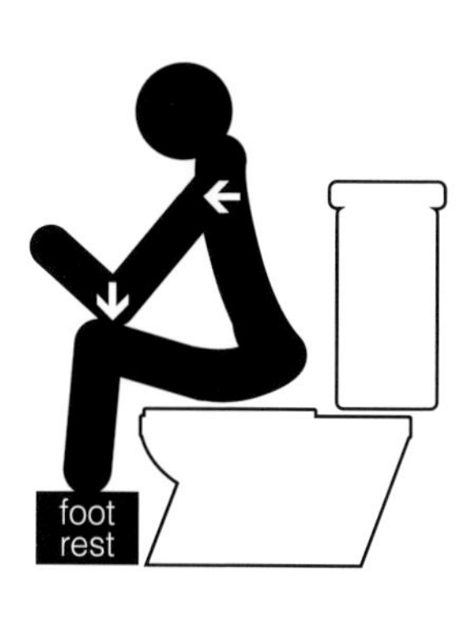

Lean forwards and put elbows on your knees

Step three

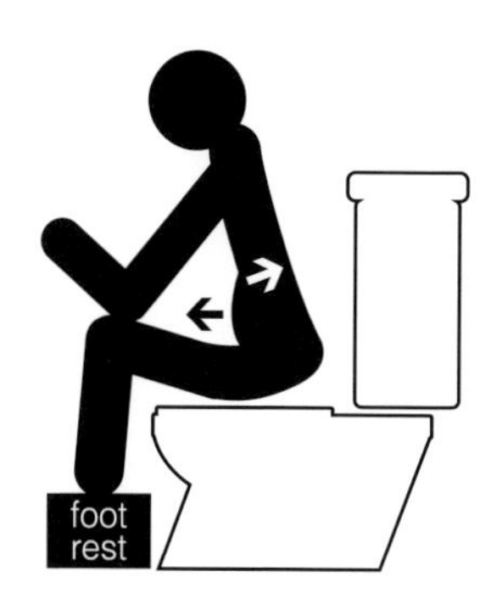

Bulge out your abdomen
Straighten your spine

Correct position

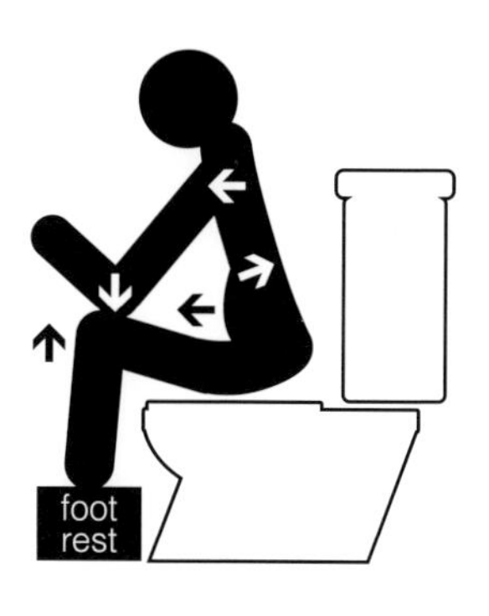

Knees higher than hips
Lean forwards and put elbows on your knees
Bulge out your abdomen
Straighten your spine

ced by the kind permission of Ray Addison, Nurse Consultant in Bladder and Bowel Dysfunction.
less, Colorectal Nurse Specialist.

d as a service to the medical profession by Norgine Ltd.

MO/03/11 (6809792) November 2003

 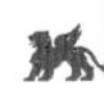

You can help ensure the pouch is empty by wiggling your hips, gently massaging the abdomen, coughing or laughing. It may be useful to stand up and then sit straight down again. If the stool is not draining, the catheter may need a flush. Attach the bladder syringe to the end of the catheter and gently flush with 20–30 ml of water. To remove, pull downwards whilst gently rolling between your fingers. The Medena™ catheter is reusable so you can wash it in soapy water and then dry.

Strictures

You may have been diagnosed as having a stricture above, within or below your pouch. This is where there is a narrowing of the bowel and the pouch may become difficult to empty. Symptoms of a stricture include pouch frequency, leakage, abdominal pain, cramping or incomplete emptying of the pouch. If it is possible to reach the stricture it may be recommended that you use a metal instrument known as a Hegar dilator to prevent it from narrowing down.

Your pouch nurse will be able to show you how to do this. Hegar dilators come in different sizes and need to be prescribed by the medical team. You will be advised how often the dilator needs to be used but it is normally once a day to stretch the narrowing. The dilator can be cleaned in warm, soapy water and then dried and kept in a safe place. If it is not possible to dilate or widen the narrowing manually then it may be necessary to have a simple operation first. You are then taught how to use a Hegar dilator.

Instructions for using a Hegar dilator

Equipment needed: Hegar dilator or St Mark's dilator, lubricating jelly or Lidocaine gel. To use the dilator:

- Ensure that your pouch is empty before using the dilator
- Insert the end of the dilator into the pot of gel or use your finger to lubricate the end of the dilator
- Lie on your left side and if possible draw your knees up to your chest.
- Insert the dilator into the anus about 3–6 cm
- The pouch nurse or doctor will be able to advise you how far you need to insert the dilator
- Rotate the dilator 360 degrees and then remove slowly

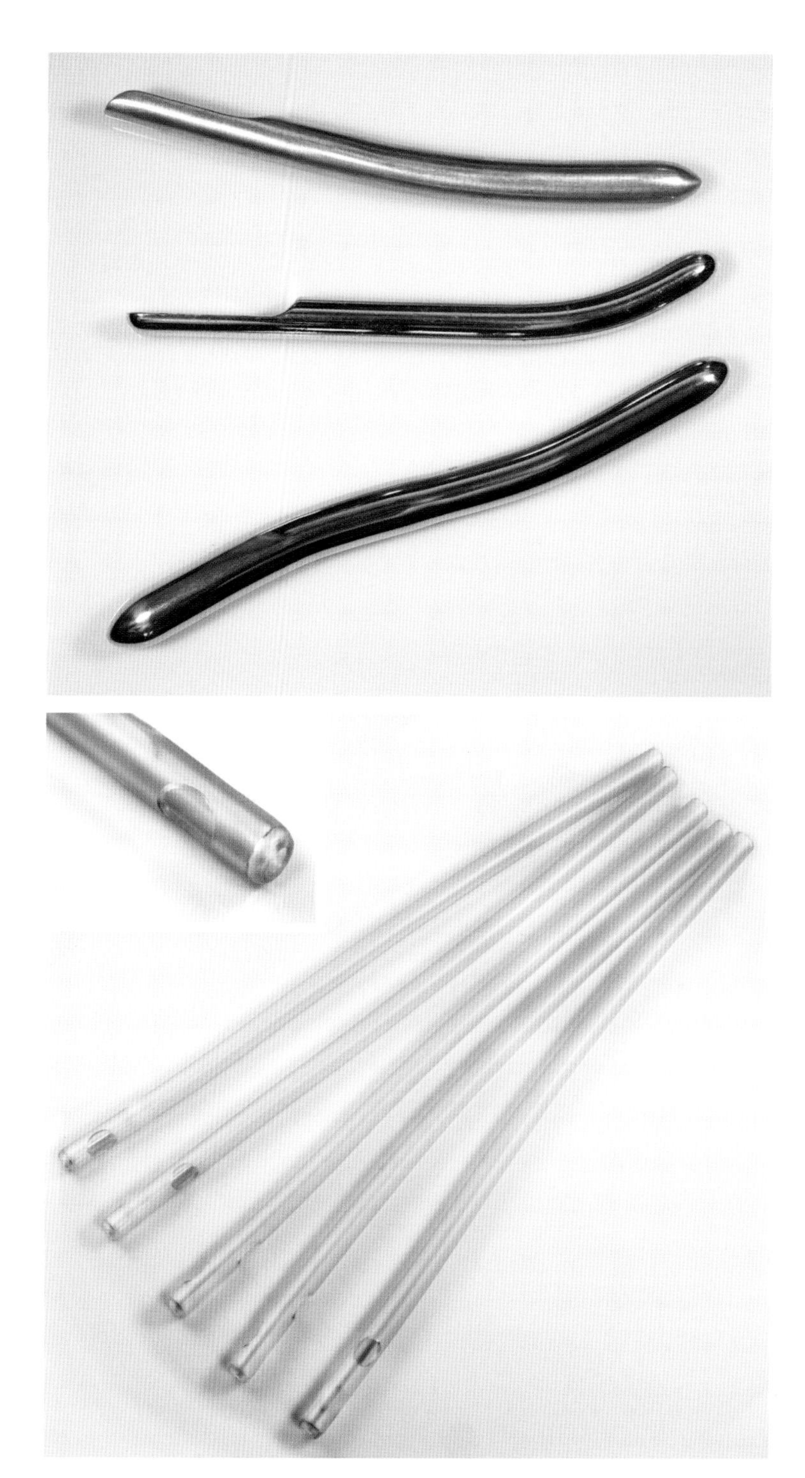

Hegar dilators and St Mark's dilators (above) and Medena™ catheters (below)

 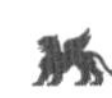

Where to get the equipment

Lidocaine 2% gel will lubricate and numb an area as it has a local anaesthetic agent in it. Lidocaine gel is only available in pots via Northwick Park and St Mark's Hospital pharmacy. You could ask your GP for a prescription which can be taken to your chemist. Your chemist can then create an account for you to get Lidocaine gel locally. The number for the pharmacy department at Northwick Park and St Mark's Hospital is 0208 869 2295 and your chemist can speak to a hospital pharmacist to discuss whether this will be possible.

A similar product to Lidocaine (Instillagel®) can be prescribed but is not as thick in consistency.

Medena™ catheters are dispensed by a company called Wellspect Health Care and are available on prescription from your GP quoting code number 68735.

Hegar dilators are available from a company called Seward Thackery. They are available as either single or double-ended dilators. Single-ended dilators are only one size whereas double-ended dilators have two different widths on the same dilator. These are available from the Northwick Park Hospital pharmacy. Alternatively, you will have to see your GP and ask your chemist to order you one. You may be able to purchase them on the internet.

Seepage: Blood, mucous, loose stool or a combination of these products may occasionally seep from the pouch without you being aware of it happening but is not always a cause of concern. If seepage of any degree continues to be a problem it is advisable to speak to a pouch nurse who will be able to guide you as to whether medication might help or if further investigation is required.

Leakage: Most people have experienced some leakage from their pouch but this usually gets better with time. Leakage can happen in the first few weeks after closure of the stoma as everything is settling down but for some people it is a continuing problem. Leakage quite commonly occurs at night when lying down and more relaxed. Some people wear a pad so that they feel a bit more secure and until they are able to manage and understand the way their pouch functions.

Incontinence occurs when you are unable to hold onto the contents of the pouch long enough to get to the toilet. This can sometimes be a problem in the first few days after stoma closure, if you have looser stool than usual, inflammation, damage to the sphincter muscles or as the pouch ages.

Pouchitis

Pouchitis is a condition where the pouch becomes inflamed. Pouchitis only occurs after closure of the stoma when the pouch is fully functioning. It can lead to symptoms of increased pouch frequency, urgency, cramping pain and occasionally bleeding and fever. This is common in people undergoing pouch surgery for ulcerative colitis. Over ten years of having a pouch, up to half the patients undergoing pouch surgery may develop a single, brief episode of pouch inflammation, which usually settles with a short course of antibiotic treatment. For a small proportion of patients the inflammation can persist requiring further antibiotics. In an even smaller proportion pouchitis can be long-standing and more difficult to treat.

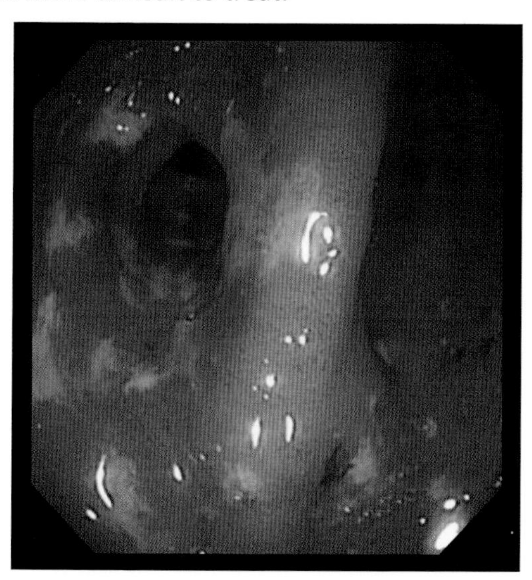

Pouchoscopy showing pouchitis

Pouchitis can often be confused with other causes of inflammation within the pouch such as poor emptying of the pouch leading to stasis of the pouch contents, drugs such as anti-inflammatory painkillers or uncommon infections. These need to be excluded.

To accurately diagnose pouchitis the symptoms mentioned above need to be present, but there also needs to be evidence of pouchitis on pouchoscopy (a camera test of the pouch – either with a flexible camera in the endoscopy department or a short telescope used in the clinic) and on biopsy samples from the lining of the pouch.

If pouchitis is confirmed it is usually treated with a two week course of antibiotics (usually Ciprofloxacin or Metronidazole). Sometimes, your doctor may suggest you take these antibiotics whilst you are awaiting further investigations to confirm the diagnosis of pouchitis, particularly if you are unwell.

Pouchitis usually settles after a course of antibiotics, but some patients whose symptoms do not resolve may require a further 28 days of treatment with two antibiotics (usually Ciprofloxacin and Metronidazole). If the pouch inflammation completely settles after 28 days of two antibiotics and there is no evidence of inflammation on pouchoscopy, some patients may benefit from a probiotic called VSL#3. This probiotic contains a large number of bacteria per dose. Some studies suggest VSL#3 may maintain remission from pouchitis in patients whose symptoms and endoscopic inflammation have completely resolved after 28 days of antibiotics, however, this is not always the case in real life and it may be worth discussing it with your doctor. You may also have to purchase VSL#3 yourself.

A small minority of patients have persistent inflammation despite treatment or their symptoms rapidly recur after stopping treatment. Other treatment options are available which may be considered by your specialist. Rarely does persistent inflammation require permanent defunctioning or removal of the pouch.

Cuffitis

Cuffitis is a term you may hear about from your doctor. It means there is inflammation in the cuff of rectum that is left to attach the pouch on to. Occasionally in patients with ulcerative colitis this can become inflamed due to ulcerative colitis recurring in this remaining rectal tissue. Symptoms may be very similar to those of pouchitis with increased frequency of opening the pouch, bleeding and pain. This can be diagnosed on pouchoscopy and biopsy of the residual cuff of rectum. Treatment usually involves topical application of medication that you may have used previously if you had ulcerative colitis such as suppositories of Mesalazine or steroid suppositories.

Pre-pouch ileitis

Pre-pouch ileitis refers to inflammation of the small bowel above the pouch. This is generally only found in some patients who also have pouchitis. It does not normally mean that there is a change in diagnosis to Crohn's disease but this was previously thought to be the case. It can often cause no symptoms and is found incidentally when assessing pouchitis with a camera test, however, it can lead to frequency, cramping pain and occasionally blockages due to strictures of the bowel above the pouch that may require stretching during an endoscopic procedure or may require further surgery. It can be treated with antibiotics similarly to pouchitis.

Crohn's disease

Rarely inflammation can occur in the pouch that is actually considered to be due to Crohn's disease rather than pouchitis when looking at the biopsy samples that are taken. This occurs in less than 4 in 100 cases. Symptoms can be similar to those of pouchitis, but require treatment with medications for Crohn's disease or most often requires permanent defunctioning or removal of the pouch.

Irritable pouch syndrome

The symptoms of frequency, urgency and pain can also occur in patients with no evidence of inflammation of the pouch when assessed by pouchoscopy and biopsies. It is not well understood, but it is considered that a syndrome similar to irritable bowel syndrome can also affect patients with pouches. An American study showed that 4 out of 10 patients who had symptoms of frequency, urgency and pain did not have any inflammation of the pouch. It is not clear (as for irritable bowel syndrome) why this may occur. There are no clear treatment approaches for 'irritable pouch syndrome', but treatments aimed at managing symptoms appear to be effective. These include reassurance, dietary fibre supplementation, anti-diarrhoeal and antispasmodic medication and antidepressant therapy. Antidepressant therapies are thought to be effective at very low doses, to modulate the nerves that control pouch function and sensation.

Urgency

If you experience urgency to empty your pouch it could be an indication

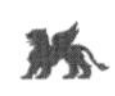

that you may have some degree of inflammation such as pouchitis or gastroenteritis or you may have an obstruction of some sort which will require investigation. If the urgency continues for more than a couple of days you should consult your pouch nurse or doctor.

Fistula

Pouch fistulae are more often seen as a late complication. A fistula occurs when a defect in the pouch creates a tract for stool to pass into the vagina or buttocks. Pouch vaginal or pouch perineal fistula occurs in 5–10% of patients with pouches created for ulcerative colitis. Sometimes the diagnosis is changed to Crohn's disease in the presence of these fistulae after investigations. Placing a seton (a loose thread through the outside defect leading into the pouch) is the treatment of choice as the alternative operation of laying open the fistula, may result in incontinence. In some circumstances it may be necessary to redo the pouch or create a permanent stoma if there is no symptomatic control with a seton.

Small volume pouch

The pouch when created is designed to act like a rectum which stores the stool before it is evacuated. A certain volume is required to ensure that the pouch provides the necessary lifestyle requirements of the pouch. A pouch that is too small can result in emptying difficulties or increased frequency. Revision surgery may be required in this situation but is not always successful.

Pouch failure

Pouch failure occurs when complications cannot be managed by conservative means and the only option is reverting to a stoma. About 10% of pouches fail over a ten year period. Pouch failure can be quite devastating as the symptoms may last for many years and can result in significant lifestyle implications. In some situations it may be possible to revise the pouch provided the operation is done by an experienced surgeon. In the situation where revision surgery is not indicated or not successful then a permanent stoma will be required. The commonest reason for failure is sepsis (50%). Another common cause for failure is poor pouch function which ultimately causes a reduced quality of life.

Pouch investigations

Unfortunately for some people, complications may arise with the pouch that warrants further investigation. If your doctor or pouch nurse thinks a test or investigation is appropriate they will arrange one and also follow up the results. This is usually done as an outpatient. Some of these tests or investigations are only performed in specialist centres where the correct equipment is available and trained and experienced staff will interpret the results. Some people may have a slightly altered pouch function for a few days after some tests but this is normal, however, if you are concerned you should seek medical advice.

A digital examination is one of the simplest tests to examine the anastomosis (join) between the pouch and anal canal and also any abnormalities inside the anus. You will be asked to lie on your left side on the examination couch with your knees drawn up towards your chest. The assessment will be performed by the pouch nurse or doctor who will insert a lubricated finger into your anus. This may be a little uncomfortable but should take less than a minute to complete. As with most investigations the more you can relax the easier the examination will become. Most of the time a digital examination will be performed before any other investigation.

Rigid pouchoscopy is used to see the quality of the lining of the pouch or gently dilate a tight anastomosis. You will be asked to empty your pouch before the examination if you are able. A rigid scope is inserted into your pouch and air is used to move the bowel so the pouch lining can be seen more clearly. This may become a little uncomfortable. If it is too painful it will be abandoned and a flexible pouchoscopy booked if necessary.

Flexible pouchoscopy is performed in the Endoscopy department to confirm or exclude inflammation, polyps or strictures. Seven days before your pouchoscopy you may have to stop medication such as Warfarin, Clopidogrel, Aspirin and iron tablets as we usually take biopsies of the pouch. You must speak to your GP or cardiologist before stopping your medication! On the day of the test you will be given an enema into the pouch to improve visibility in the pouch. You will be asked to wear a hospital gown so it may be wise to bring a dressing gown and slippers. Though you can eat and drink as normal it may be more comfortable if you have only a light meal before the test. A flexible scope is inserted into your pouch and air and water is used to move the bowel so the pouch can be seen clearly. Biopsies are taken of the pouch lining and cuff. This may cause a little bleeding which is normal. You will be able to see the test being done on a screen in front of you if you wish. Some patients may experience an erratic pouch function for 24–48 hours afterwards. If the test is uncomfortable you may be offered a smaller scope or mild sedation. You may also be offered pain relief. If you have sedation it is recommended that you have assistance getting home as you will not be able to drive a car or use public transport alone. You will then have an outpatient appointment or telephone consultation in approximately two weeks to discuss your results.

A pouchogram is routinely performed to check for leakage between the pouch and anal canal prior to stoma closure, however, it can also be used to detect any leaks or fistulae in the pouch or anal canal. No preparation is required and you can eat and drink as normal on the day. You will be asked to wear a hospital gown so it may be wise to bring a dressing gown and slippers. Whilst lying on your side on the table, a medium-sized catheter is lubricated and then inserted into the pouch. It is taped onto your bottom so it does not fall out. We mix 100 ml of Gastrografin® fluid and 300 ml of water in an irrigation bag. This bag is suspended on a stand and the fluid flows into your pouch via the catheter. The table is tilted and a series of X-rays are taken as you are rolled gently into different positions. This takes about fifteen minutes. The fluid is then allowed to drain out of the catheter once the test is complete. You will be given a pad and disposable underwear as it is possible that the Gastrografin® fluid will drain out when you start walking. This test involves X-rays and the usual precautions are taken.

A defaecating pouchogram is used to assess functional problems within the pouch such as incomplete emptying. There is no preparation required and you can eat and drink as usual before the test. You will be asked to wear a hospital gown so it may be wise to bring a dressing gown and slippers. Three 50 ml bladder syringes are prepared, one with a barium paste and the other two with barium liquid.

You will be asked to lie on your side and then a lubricated syringe tip is inserted into your anus to introduce the barium into the pouch. You are then seated onto a mini-commode behind a screen and asked to evacuate the pouch.

Though this is not a dignified test it is very diagnostic and helpful in assessing what may be wrong with your pouch. It is completed in fifteen minutes. You will be given a pad and disposable underwear as it is possible that the barium will drain out when you start walking. This test involves X-rays and the usual precautions are taken.

Examination under anaesthetic (EUA) is performed under general anaesthetic in theatre. You are put to sleep so that the surgeon can examine your pouch effectively, especially if it is too uncomfortable to do so when you are awake. Biopsies and a pouchoscopy may be done at the same time.

Anal physiology or manometry is used to see how the muscles and nerves around the anal canal work. Usually a very small catheter with a balloon on the end is inserted into the anus and measurements are taken. The test takes about fifteen minutes, however, you will be asked a series of questions to ascertain your pouch function before the test starts. It should not be painful but if your anal canal is sore it may be a little uncomfortable.

Biofeedback is a combination of behavioural therapies used to retrain the bowel and associated muscles. It is performed over a series of visits with a specialist biofeedback nurse. Sometimes anal physiology is requested before biofeedback starts. This service is not offered in all hospitals.

Magnetic resonance imaging (MRI) is performed in the X-ray department but without the use of X-rays. It is usually performed to see what is happening outside or around your pouch. You lie in a MRI scanner which consists of a large and very strong magnet and then radio waves are passed over your abdomen and pelvis. These returning signals are converted into pictures by a computer attached to the scanner. An MRI is quite safe in the majority of patients unless you have metal implants.

The results of any investigations will be discussed in clinic. It may also be possible to discuss some results and make management plans for you over the phone with your pouch nurse.

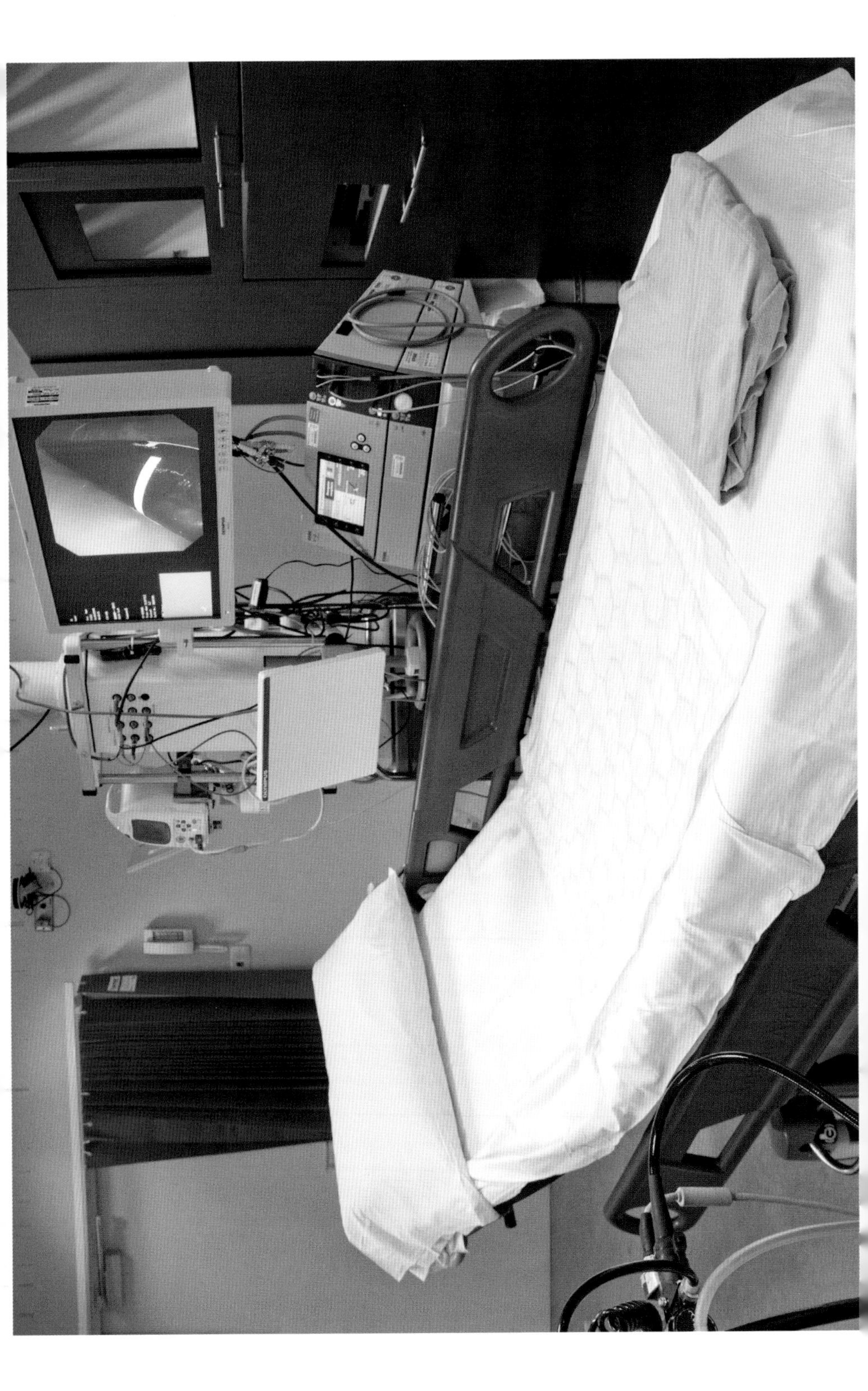

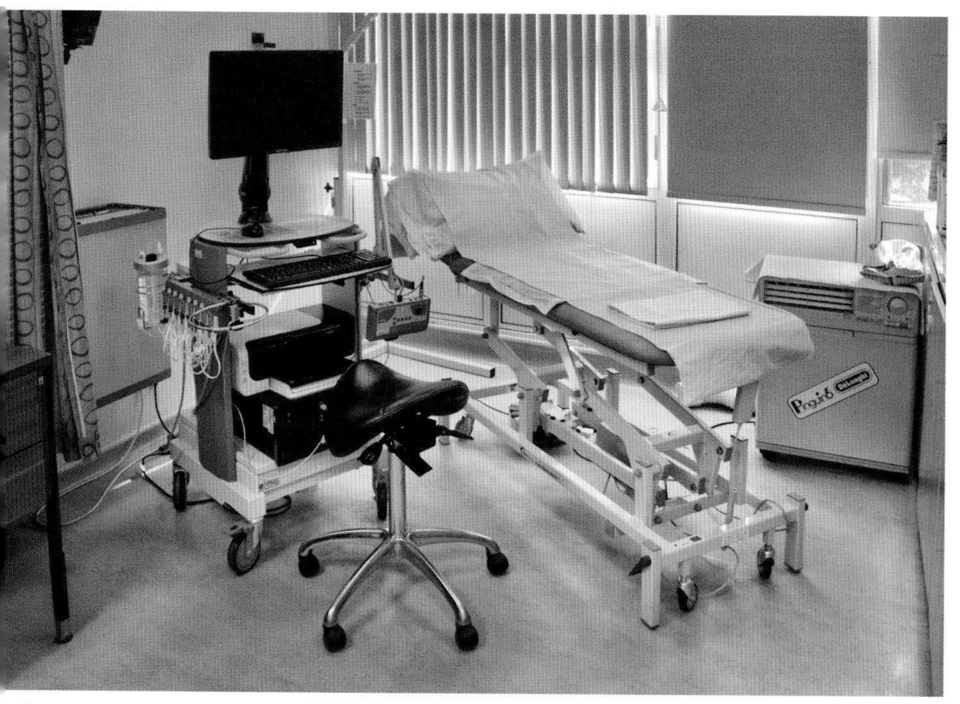

above: manometry station and patient bed

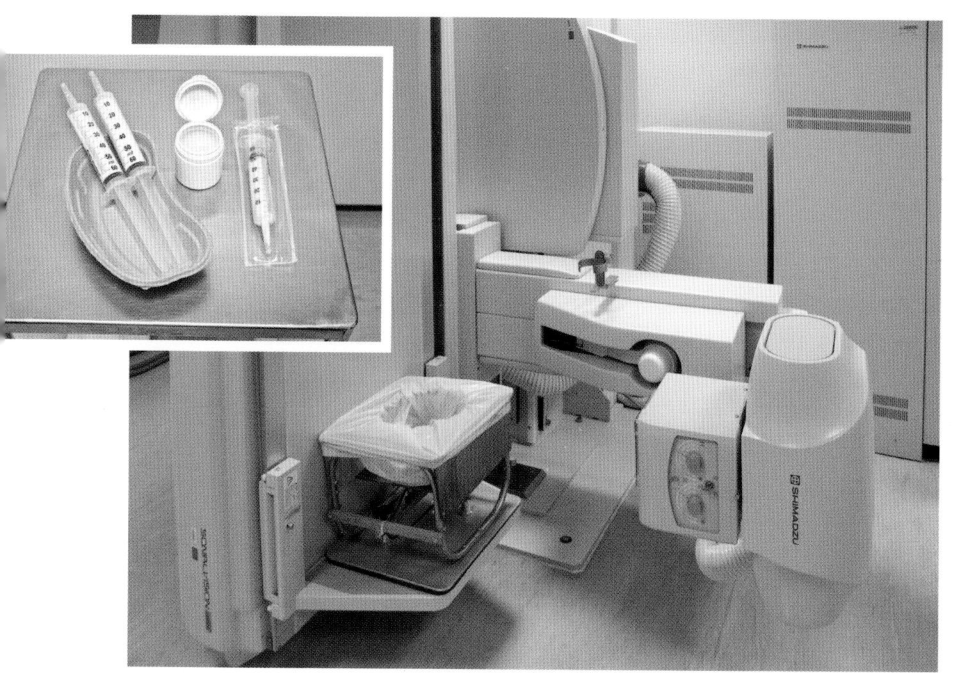

above: a mini-commode; inset: pre-filled syringes with barium

Patient experience

Rio Diedrick

Age at time of surgery: 17–25 years
Sex: female
Diagnosis: UC
First operation: emergency
Type of operation: open surgery
Number of operations: 3 stages

Life with a stoma

As the surgery wasn't planned and I had little time to get to grips with what was going on I found it hard initially to cope with my stoma. Being 20 at the time I had my first stage, I worried about the thought of having a stoma for the rest of my life and what others might think of me. It completely knocked my confidence and self-esteem. Over a period of several months, however, my confidence grew and I became comfortable with the bag. Not long after, I had the second stage of the pouch surgery and had a temporary loop ileostomy. Whilst my end stoma gave me no physical problems this was not the same with the loop. I had a high output which caused problems with dehydration and a flush stoma which caused problems with my skin. As I knew the loop ileostomy was only temporary though, I managed the problems with loperamide, convex bags and barrier creams. It was reversed five months later.

Life with a pouch

I was prepared for a long journey with my pouch and knew it wouldn't be an easy ride initially. It took some time getting used to my 'new plumbing'. After three months with the pouch I started to have increased frequency, pain, I was passing blood and just generally felt unwell. My symptoms were diagnosed as pouchitis, which was later confirmed with a scope, so I was given a course of antibiotics. After this, my pouch went from strength to strength. Over eighteen months I noticed a remarkable difference in my pouch function and my overall health. I could pretty much eat what I wanted and do what I wanted. I slowly started to think less and less about my pouch as it didn't restrict me in any way. Whilst there were times I thought I'd made the wrong choice overall my recovery went well and three years down the line I am happy with my decision.

Support I received

My support came from my stoma nurse and the IA (The Ileostomy & Internal Pouch Support Group). My stoma nurse provided me with lots of support within the first few weeks but after that I felt like I was alone. I was told I could call her at any time but didn't feel I was able to contact her for minor things. I contacted IA and referred myself to their visiting service and was contacted by someone who also had a pouch. It was great to get firsthand knowledge from someone who already had a pouch and could answer any questions I had.

Expectations of surgery

I actually had lower expectations for my pouch surgery. The first stage of my surgery I had postoperative complications which hindered my recovery. Going into the second and third stages I thought there could be complications again and was prepared for the worst. Again, with the recovery after the final stage I had heard it takes a long time for the pouch to settle and was prepared for this. Whilst it did take eighteen months for my pouch to get to the stage where it is now, it wasn't as bad as I was expecting initially.

David Danciger

Age at time of surgery: 26–36 years
Sex: male
Diagnosis: UC
First operation: emergency
Type of operation: laparoscopic (keyhole)
Number of operations: 3 stages (required an extra open surgery operation due to a complication three weeks after the first)

Life with a stoma

It was very difficult. The stoma was always on my mind and the thought that it might leak. It was very time consuming and unpleasant to deal with. I did get used to it though I was never happy. I did not go to any crowded places and was not myself the whole time.

The loop stoma was even more difficult to maintain. I had to use a special bag and didn't wear normal clothes, just tracksuit bottoms.

If you are young, active and energetic then life with a stoma isn't really a life at all.

Life with a pouch

I was lucky my pouch adapted quickly. Within a month I was down to 6–8 hours in every 24 hours. Was back in the gym six weeks after surgery. I still didn't fully recover my energy until about six months later.

It's very time consuming, I probably spend one and a half hours a day in the toilet due to a stricture. I am still on two loperamide a day but this is now part of life and you can do other stuff whilst on the toilet!

I have to be strategic when eating and now tolerate using toilets that I would never have done before but have not let this stop me doing anything over the past six months. This has been one of the best periods of my life. I'm able to play football, travel lots and have probably had way too much alcohol.

I have to be careful as the skin still gets a bit sore, but I hardly need to use any cream anymore and as long as I use quality toilet paper there isn't a problem.

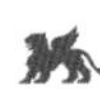

Support I received

My parents and my pouch nurse were always available if needed.

Expectations of surgery

Before the first surgery I had no idea things would be as bad when recovering, for example, suffering from ileus, wound infections, having to force myself to learn how to eat again and the time it took to recover. I was really looking forward to the final surgery. I couldn't wait to start the final recovery. Now I'm very happy with the outcome.

Other comments

I had a number of complications, it was extremely tough but if you have the right support and attitude you can get through it. Based on how my life is now I would have elected to have the surgeries given the choice.

I was unlucky with complications, most people won't be. Now I feel like I have a new lease of life and it's great!

John Mullins

Age at time of surgery: 37–47 years
Sex: male
Diagnosis: UC
First operation: planned
Type of operation: open
Number of operations: 2 stages

Life with a stoma

I had a stoma for six months. As my surgery was planned I was fortunate enough to be well prepared for life with an ileostomy. I had managed to speak with a number of people about what to expect and as a result had no real shocks when I came around after surgery. I had a very supportive stoma care nurse who taught me well about taking care of the stoma.

I was warned loop ileostomies could be quite troublesome but I didn't seem to have any problems that others hadn't already had. I did have a couple of leaks, a supportive and understanding partner and a good sense of humour made dealing with them much easier. All in all I found life with a stoma much easier than I expected, so much so that I considered not going through with my final surgery. Being healthy again made a huge contribution to these feelings, my life was so much better than it had been and I was worried that might change after the final surgery. It wasn't until my sick colon had been removed that I realised just how ill UC had made me.

Life with a pouch

It is now close on twelve years since my final surgery and it is probably fair to say I have had a good result. Initially I took things very slowly, being very careful with what I ate and drank. Over time, foods I was wary of have been reincorporated back into my diet and now I do not give what I eat a second thought, this is probably a good thing as food and drink are one of my passions. I have excellent pouch function and toilet visits are much fewer than I was expecting and I usually sleep through the night.

When I was ill, keeping fit was never really an option, I never had the energy. Since my surgery it has almost become essential, UC always left me underweight but now I am healthy again I put on weight very easily.

To keep this in check I started swimming and attending my local gym and more recently I have taken up road cycling.

When I was ill, we were always a little wary of travel and this limited how often we visited new places, however, since surgery we have no such worries and are slowly but surely ticking the boxes on our bucket list of places to visit.

I have had the misfortune to have a few bouts of pouchitis but these have always been cleared up with a course of antibiotics and have only caused me issues for a few days at a time. I have viewed these few days of discomfort a fair swap for the remaining twelve years of good health and would make that deal again tomorrow. It is very rare that I think about my surgery now and never really give my pouch a second thought.

Support I received

My pouch nurse was my primary point of support, always on hand to answer my questions and put my mind at ease when I had problems – twelve years on and we are still friends. She put me in touch with IA who introduced me to others who had been through surgery and could share their experiences with me which was a huge help. Meeting others and seeing they were now just fit and healthy, normal people was a great source of comfort going into surgery. My employers were helpful giving me all the time off I needed and working with me to get back to a normal working life as soon as possible after both surgeries.

Expectations of surgery

My only real hopes of surgery were to be healthy again. I understood that life might not be perfect but after suffering with UC for such a long time I was prepared to make the compromises that were needed in exchange for being well once more. I have been fortunate enough that no real compromises have been needed and my life after surgery has far exceeded any expectations.

Other comments

The support I received from my medical team and the patient organisations was invaluable and I would recommend anybody going through this surgery to seek out the same support. It made my recovery so much easier than it might otherwise have been.

Bharat Bhushan Sharma

Age at time of surgery: 47–67 years
Sex: male
Diagnosis: UC
First operation: planned
Type of operation: open surgery
Number of operations: 3 stages

Life with a stoma

I had a stoma twice. The first time around, life with the stoma was terrible.

The spout of my stoma was more or less flush with my abdomen and the stoma used to leak a lot. I would get up in the middle of night to find all my night-suit and the bed linen soiled. I had to get up and clean myself and have a shower in the middle of the night. I was always scared to go out in case my stoma leaked. On one occasion it did and was a very embarrassing moment for me. All this happened because I was overweight before my operation which made my surgery difficult. My surgeon told me that he was not going to operate on me for second stage unless I lost 25% of my body weight, which I managed to lose with the help of a very nice, dedicated and helpful pouch nurse. I had my reversal and had a stoma for about nine months and this time around the stoma worked fine and I began to feel comfortable with my stoma.

Life with a pouch

I had a pouch for about five years and it was like having UC all over again. It was mostly okay in the beginning and after a few months of having a pouch, I was having stomach cramps and urgency to go to the toilet.

There were times when I was going to toilet eleven or twelve times a day and it felt at times that I was spending half a day in the toilet.

If I went out, I was looking for the toilet most of the time and if I did not find one in time I would suffer with a lot of stomach pains and urgency.

I could not travel by bus on long journeys because of my dysfunctional pouch. Doctors and nurses tried all the medication which was available for my

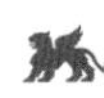

condition but nothing worked. I suffered for five long years hoping that may be there will be some cure for this.

I did not want to have a stoma again because of the previous experience I had with a stoma. There was nothing doctors or nurses could do for me.

I had to agree to have a stoma because life with a pouch was just unbearable. Fortunately, I have had a stoma now for nearly a year, it is a good stoma with a nice spout and I have had no problems with it.

Support I received

I have had support from my pouch nurse but may have needed more help, maybe?

Expectations of surgery

I was expecting to be normal after my pouch, that was the reason I decided to have a pouch initially. Unfortunately it was not meant to be.

Other comments

I am very fortunate to have been treated in St Mark's Hospital. St Mark's has the best doctors and surgeons and very helpful, dedicated pouch nurses.

I thank them from the bottom of my heart with all the help and support they gave me during my treatment.

Preash Lad

Age at time of surgery: 17–25 years
Sex: male
Diagnosis: UC
First operation: planned privately
Type of operation: laparoscopic (keyhole)
Number of operations: 1 stage (no stoma)

Life with a pouch

Life is better than before as I can hold on and no longer need to make a mad dash! However my outputs can vary between 5–10 times a day and once at night. I generally eat and drink what I want but perhaps have got a bit complacent and should try eating recommended pouch foods.

I have had a couple bouts of pouchitis which seems to improve with VSL#3 probiotics. I take approximately ten loperamide tablets a day and Buscopan when needed.

My pouch rumbles quite a bit which can be annoying.

Support I received

My support comes from family, friends, the pouch nurse and the surgeon. I was lucky to have had all of that.

Expectations of surgery

I was pretty positive that it would work. I was hoping for less outputs a day – perhaps 2–4 times and also to not be on any medication.

Other comments

I have my life back (not that the UC stopped it) but I no longer have to plan around toilets!

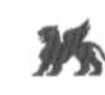

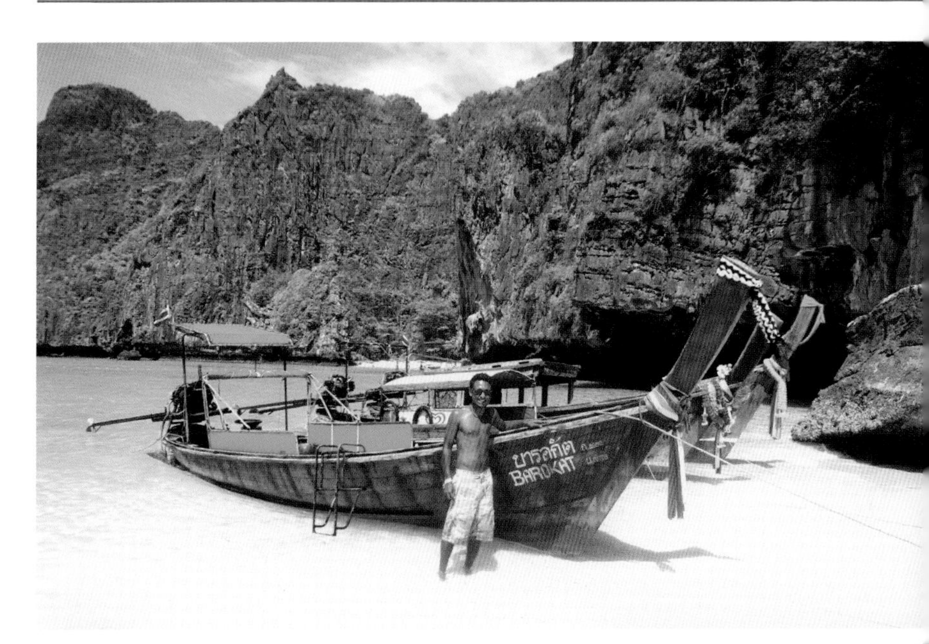

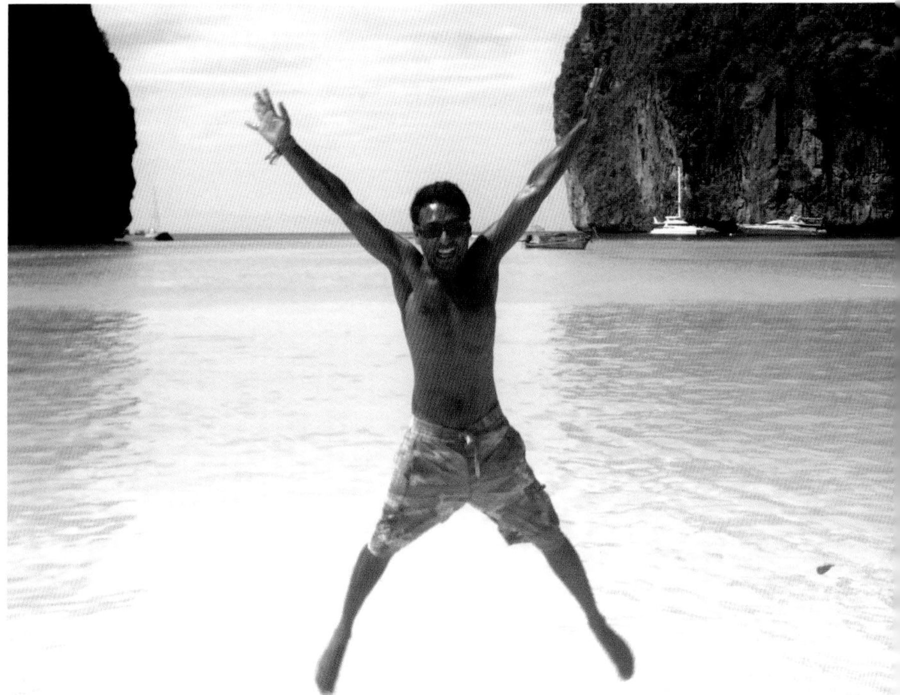

Preash Lad enjoying an overseas holiday

Support groups

Most people considering pouch surgery find it useful to talk to other people who have undergone the operation and are now living with either a pouch or stoma.

The pouch nurse and medical teams will be able to offer therapeutic advice but not be in the best position to explain the everyday lived experience. All groups have an up-to-date website, while some allow interactive chat rooms or advice lines.

For those who like face-to-face meetings these can also be arranged through some groups. Open days and sponsored events are usually offered to members and non-members and it is worthwhile having a look at different websites.

Patients who are well-informed and prepared for their pouch surgery are usually the ones who deal with this life-changing operation better.

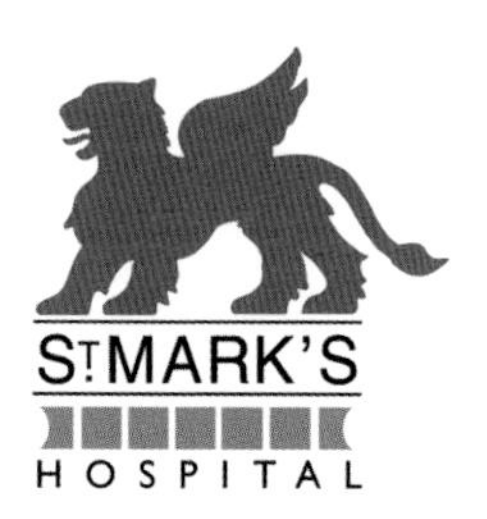

Tel: 0208 235 4126
E-Mail: lnwh-tr.internalpouchcare@nhs.net
Web: www.stmarkshospital.nhs.uk

St Mark's Hospital is the largest centre for ileo-anal pouches in the UK with six consultant surgeons performing both open and laparoscopic pouch surgery within the NHS and privately. The pouch team at St Mark's Hospital are always on hand to offer support not only to inpatients or outpatients of the hospital but anyone with a pouch or who is considering one.

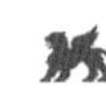

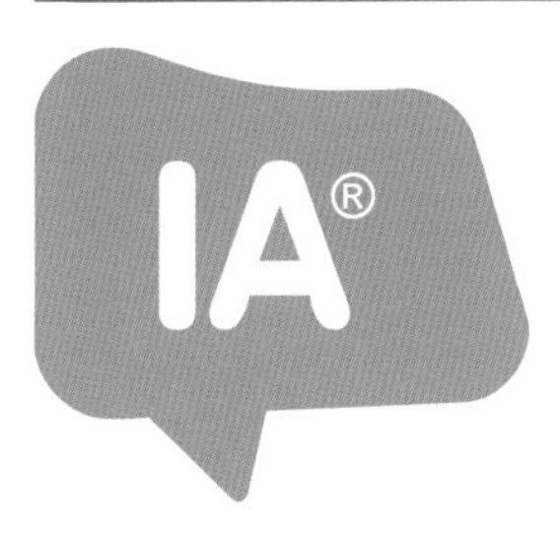

Tel: 0800 0184 724
E-Mail: info@iasupport.org
Web: www.iasupport.org

IA – the Ileostomy and Internal Pouch Support Group – is a UK registered charity whose primary aim is to help people who have to undergo surgery which involves the removal of their colon (known as a colectomy) and the creation of either an ileostomy or an ileo-anal pouch.

CROHN'S & COLITIS UK

Tel: 01727 830038
E-Mail: enquiries@crohnsandcolitis.org.uk
Web: www.nacc.org.uk

The National Association for Crohn's and Colitis (NACC) Crohn's and Colitis UK aims to improve life for everyone affected by Inflammatory Bowel Disease (IBD), the most common forms being Crohn's Disease and Ulcerative Colitis. Together these conditions affect about 250,000 people in the United Kingdom. The charity brings together people of all ages who have been diagnosed with IBD, their families and the health professionals involved in their care.

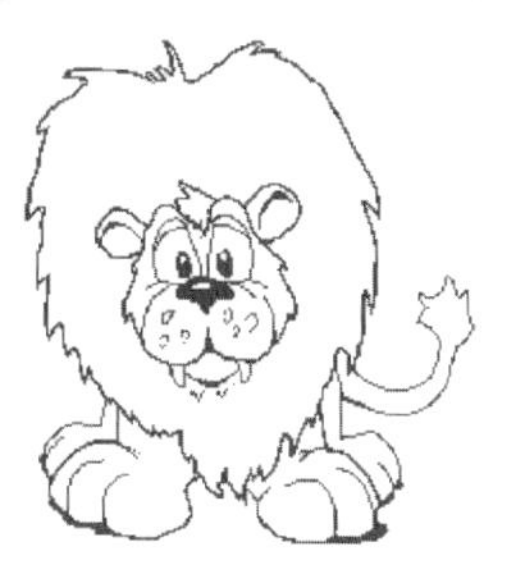

E-Mail: liaison@redliongroup.org
Web: www.redliongroup.org

The Red Lion Group is a UK pouch support charity for people who have or are considering having an ileo-anal pouch. The pouch support group was founded in 1994 by a group of patients and staff at St Mark's Hospital in London and gained charitable status in 1997. We publish a newsletter called Roar! two or three times a year and meet once a year at an Information Day to hear guest speakers and take part in group seminars covering topics of interest to pouch owners and prospective pouch owners.

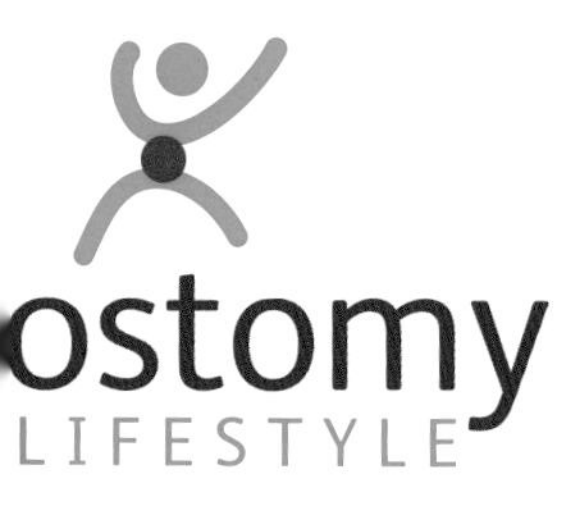

Tel: 0800 731 4264 or 01183 240089
E-Mail: advice@ostomylifestyle.org
Web: www.ostomylifestyle.org

Ostomy Lifestyle is a UK charity established in 2007 to provide support, advice and information to anyone affected by surgery to the bowel or bladder.

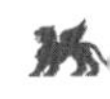

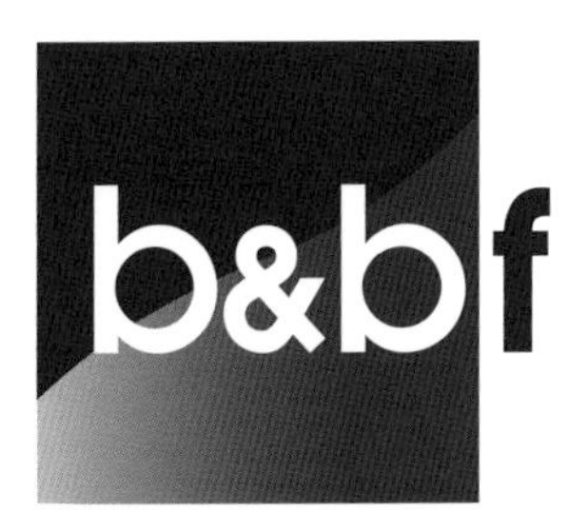

Tel: 0845 345 0165
E-Mail: info@bladderandbowelfoundation.org
Web: www.bladderandbowelfoundation.org

The Bladder and Bowel Foundation or B&BF is a UK-wide charity that provides information and advice on a range of symptoms and conditions related to the bladder and bowel.

Gay and Lesbian Ostomates

Web: www.glo-uoa.org

Although any ostomist is very welcome to view this site, gay, bi, transgender or just 'gay friendly', I'm sure you will find it both interesting and informative. The aim of this website is to provide you with news about events, products, health information in a friendly format and the chance to e-mail each other and possibly meet up with the hope that life can be improved for many who often feel very isolated at times.

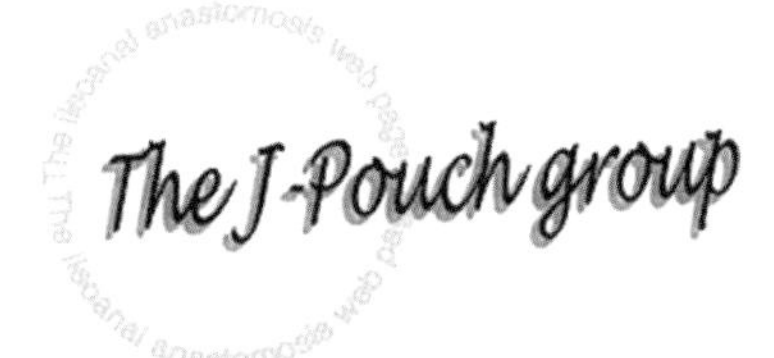

Web: www.j-pouch.org

An American website for interactive support and information regarding this procedure. The site offers a wealth of information as you plan for the operation or are dealing with life after suffering with ulcerative colitis, cancer or familial polyposis.

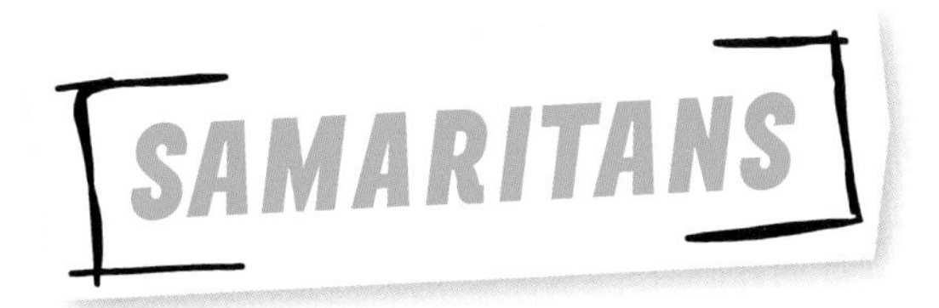

Tel: 08457 90 90 90 for the UK
Tel: 1850 60 90 90 for the Rep. of Ireland
E-Mail: Samaritans at jo@samaritans.org
Web: http://www.samaritans.org

The Samaritans is a confidential, emotional support service for anyone in the UK and Ireland. The service is available 24 hours a day for people who are experiencing feelings of distress or despair, including those which may lead to suicide. If you live outside of the UK and Republic of Ireland, visit www.befrienders.org to find your nearest helpline. If you are deaf or hard of hearing, use the single national minicom number 08457 90 91 92. The address to write to is: Chris, PO Box 9090, Stirling, FK8 2SA

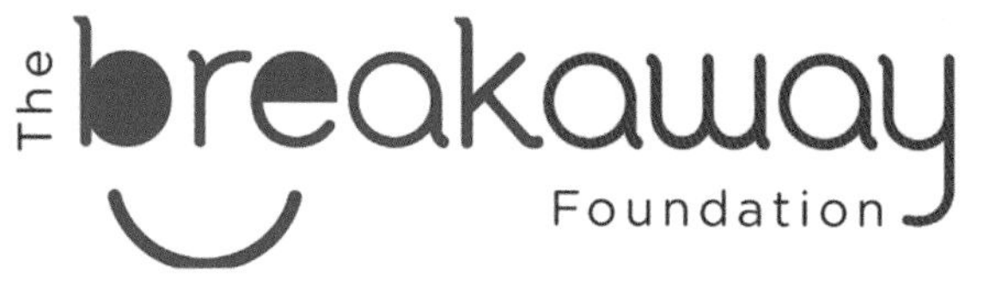

Tel: 01283 240253
E-Mail: info@breakawayfoundation.org.uk
Web: www.breakawayfoundation.org.uk

Breakaway are the UK's only weekend activity breaks designed for young people from 4–18 years old with bowel and/or bladder dysfunctions and their families. Weekends are devised and organised by people with a full knowledge of living with a bowel or bladder dysfunction. Breakaway weekends and events offer a unique opportunity for families and young people in similar situations to meet, talk about and share their experiences, take part in confidence-building, action-adventure activities in a relaxed and friendly environment.

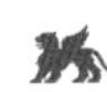

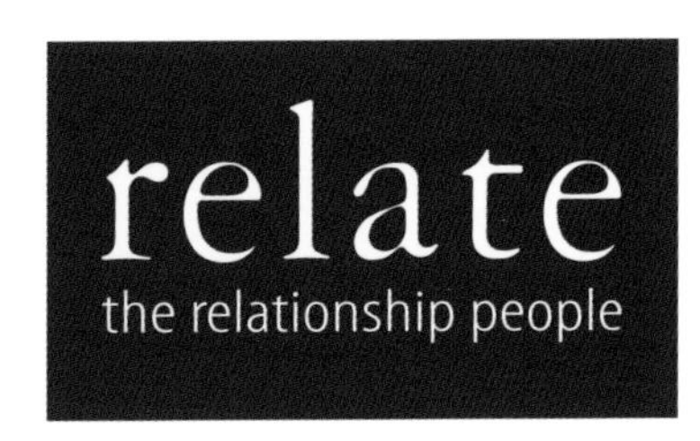

Tel: 0300 100 1234
Web: www.relate.org.uk

Relate offers psychosexual counselling through many of their local offices.